Beginning Again

D1018250

Beginning Again

Benedictine Wisdom for Living with Illness

Mary C. Earle

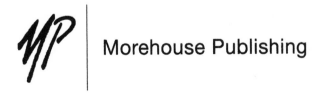

an explorefaith.org book

Morehouse Publishing

Copyright © 2004 by Mary C. Earle

All rights reserved. No part of this book may be reproduced, stored in a retrieval system, or transmitted in any form or by any means, electronic or mechanical, including photocopying, recording, or otherwise, without the written permission of the publisher.

Unless otherwise noted the Scripture quotations herein are from the New Revised Standard Version of the Bible, copyright © 1989 by the Division of Christian Education of the National Council of Churches of Christ in the U.S.A. Used by permission. All rights reserved.

"The Road Ahead" from *Thoughts in Solitude* by Thomas Merton. Copyright © 1958 by the Abbey of Our Lady of Gethsemani. Copyright renewed 1986 by the Trustees of the Thomas Merton Legacy Trust. Reprinted by permission of Farrar, Straus and Giroux, LLC and of Curtis Brown, Ltd.

Morehouse Publishing, 4775 Linglestown Road, Harrisburg, PA 17112
Morehouse Publishing, 445 Fifth Avenue, New York, NY 10016
Morehouse Publishing is an imprint of Church Publishing Incorporated.

Cover art: Roger Allyn Lee / Superstock

Cover design by Laurie Westhafer

Library of Congress Cataloging-in-Publication Data
Earle, Mary C.
  Beginning again : Benedictine wisdom for living with illness / by Mary C. Earle.
    p. cm.
  Includes bibliographical references.
  ISBN 10 : 0-8192-1965-7
  ISBN 13 : 978-0-8192-1965-7
  1. Chronically ill--Religious life. 2. Benedict, Saint, Abbot of Monte Cassino. Regula I. Title.
  BV4910.E27 2004
  248.8'61--dc22   2004001378

Printed in the United States of America

08 09 10 11 12   6 5 4 3 2

For Mom and Dad

For Doug, Bryan, and Jason, who helped me to begin again.

And for all who have had to begin again because of illness.

Contents

Acknowledgments

This book began to insist on being written while I was in the middle of writing its predecessor, *Broken Body, Healing Spirit.* Thanks go to Debra Farrington, my editor, who as a writer understands that sometimes a new proposal comes in the midst of unfinished work. She accepted another proposal with good humor and enthusiasm. Thanks also to the various members of the classes I have taught at my parish, St. Mark's Episcopal Church in San Antonio, and at the Episcopal Seminary of the Southwest in Austin. Those students have been my teachers, and much of this material first began to take root in conversations in class.

My husband, Doug, has been my coach, my friend, my companion. He read and critiqued the text, and he helps me keep my rule.

explorefaith.org books:
An Introduction

The book you hold in your hand says a lot about you. It reflects your yearning to forge a deep and meaningful relationship with God, to open yourself to the countless ways we can experience the holy, to embrace an image of the divine that frees your soul and fortifies your heart. It is a book published with the spiritual pilgrim in mind through a collaboration of Morehouse Publishing and the Web site explorefaith.org.

The pilgrim's path cannot be mapped beforehand. It moves toward the sacred with twists and turns unique to you alone. Explorefaith.org books honor the truth that we all discover the holy through different doorways, at different points in our lives. These books offer tools for your travels—resources to help you follow your soul's purest longings. Although their approach will change, their purpose remains constant. Our hope is that they will help clear the way for you, providing fruitful avenues for experiencing God's unceasing devotion and perfect love.

www.explorefaith.org
Spiritual guidance
for anyone seeking a path to God

A non-profit Web site aimed at anyone interested in exploring spiritual issues, explorefaith.org provides an open, non-judgmental, private place for exploring your faith and deepening your connection to the sacred. Material on the site is rich and varied, created to highlight the wisdom of diverse faith traditions, while at the same time expressing the conviction that through Jesus Christ we can experience the heart of God. Tools for meditating with music, art, and poetry; essays about the spiritual meaning in popular books and first-run films; a daily devotional meditation; informative and challenging responses to questions we have all pondered; excerpts from publications with a spiritual message—all this and more is available online at explorefaith.org. As stated on the site's "Who We Are" page, explorefaith.org is deeply committed to the ongoing spiritual formation of people of all ages and all backgrounds, living in countries around the world. The simple goal is to help visitors navigate their journey in faith by providing rich and varied material about God, faith, and spirituality. That material focuses on a God of grace and compassion, whose chief characteristic is love.

You have the book, now try the Web site. Visit us at www.explorefaith.org. With its emphasis on God's infinite grace and the importance of experiencing the sacred, its openness and respect for different denominations and religions, and its grounding in the love of God expressed through Christianity, explorefaith.org can become a valued part of your faith-formation and on-going spiritual practice.

PART I

"Giving the Mess Some Meaning"

1
Introduction

I t is September 1995. Home from the hospital, I am trying to figure out who in the world I am now. I have survived the initial crisis of an attack of acute pancreatitis. I stay in bed most of the day. I very slowly gain some strength. Some days I can eat without ill effect. Some days I cannot. Every pattern to which I have been accustomed has been completely disrupted. Before the pancreatitis I was a healthy, active, engaged woman—a wife, a mother, an Episcopal priest, a spiritual director, a writer. In a matter of hours all of those identities were turned inside out and upside down as the acute pancreatitis kidnapped my life as I knew it.

When pancreatitis moved through my life like an earthquake, the recovery period left me sufficiently weakened that I found it difficult or impossible to keep the established patterns of my own spiritual practices. I was accustomed to doing yoga, keeping a journal, reading scripture, and praying every morning. At the age of forty-six, I had also begun paying attention to nutrition, exercise, and leisure as part of my own intentional plan for living. All of this was shattered by the acute illness. I barely had the energy to lie on the couch and watch a movie, much less get up and pray. Much of my waking life was dedicated to a daily education about nutrition and the difficulties of living with a weakened pancreas. (My doctor had said, "Of all the organs in the body, the pancreas is the most mysterious. We really don't know exactly how it works.")

In those first months of recovery it felt as if my life were over. I had a lot of grieving to do, grieving for a life that was lost and for a body that was afflicted. I also succumbed to the prevalent cultural notion that once illness has visited like an unwelcome guest and has, in fact, changed from being a guest to a resident, your life is over. On the one hand, this is true. The life I had once lived was now irrevocably changed. My seemingly endless energy had evaporated like dew in the sun. My omnivorous appetite had to be confined to the simplest of diets, the smallest of portions, and even then I would often break out in a cold sweat from the labor involved in digestion.

It seemed that a life with boundless horizons had been reduced to a life of one limitation after another. Some days I felt as if I were turning over rocks in a dried-up streambed, looking for signs of life, only to discover more rocks. The fact that the ailment was pancreatitis made things more difficult in some ways. "Pancreatitis" is hardly a household word. I had to educate myself about the illness, about the recovery, about the chronic aspects of the ailment. When I was in the emergency room and the doctor informed me that I had acute pancreatitis, I had to ask where the pancreas was. I had hardly been aware that I had a pancreas, much less that its malfunction could create so much havoc.

All of these limitations affected not only me but also my whole family. My husband, Doug, had to assume many of the household duties. A good cook, he had to learn what I could eat and how it had to be prepared. He, too, lost his life as he knew it. A lot had to be renegotiated in terms of the marriage. On the one hand, the words "for better and for worse, in sickness and in health" took on a depth of meaning we'd not had to know before the illness. On the other one, the daily discovery of my own real weakness caused us both stress and distress.

I had to drop out of a doctoral program in which I was enrolled and curtail many activities. Travels, retreats, teaching opportunities—all had to be forsaken. As the months passed, the weakness deepened as I continued to lose weight. CT scans, ultrasounds, and blood tests did not show evidence of malignancy. Finally, we discovered that my body was failing to metabolize my food. Though I was eating, my body was not absorbing the nutrients. I was losing weight, my skin and hair were drying out, my vision was blurring. I'd managed to develop a vitamin deficiency because of the malabsorption difficulty.

Many of you who are reading this book have suffered far worse than I. Many of you have lived with people whose lives have been completely altered by illness in one of its acute, chronic, or progressive forms. You know that living *with* illness is the reality. The illness is not likely to disappear. In fact, it becomes a major defining force in daily life. The illness comes with limitations and distress, with diminishments and loss. In the predominant culture of the United States, this is often construed to mean that whatever life might look like with illness, it is not lively. Nor is it creative. The possibility that it offers strange gifts under the guise of limitation is unimaginable. And it *certainly* could not be spiritual! Such are the prevailing misconceptions in our culture.

Living with Illness and a Rule of Life

For years before becoming ill, I lived with a simple rule of life. A rule of life, a simple monastic concept, helps us to become more mindful of divine presence throughout the day, in all persons and in all circumstances. The word "rule" is derived from the Latin word *regula*. It connotes guidance and wisdom rather than a rigid code. To follow a rule is to walk "in a path of life" (Psalm 16:11). A rule, like a path of life, is adopted and learned over time. It is not internalized all at once. It requires steadily putting one foot in front of the other (at least metaphorically) in order to reach the destination.

My own pre-illness rule of life was influenced by both the Cursillo movement and by the Rule of Saint Benedict. The former, a renewal movement that emphasizes a life marked by prayer, study, and action, began to have an effect on me after I attended a Cursillo weekend in 1979. At roughly the same time, I became aware of the Rule of Saint Benedict, an ancient rule of life dating from the sixth century. This rule, or guide for Christian living, emphasizes a life marked by prayer, holy reading, and manual labor, with vows of stability, obedience, and ongoing transformation and conversion. The Rule of Benedict is grounded in the practice of listening deeply to God and to all of life. Benedict also invites us to prefer nothing to Christ. With common sense and gentleness, Benedict provides for life in community that respects the young, the ill, and the elderly. His is a vision of shared life in Christ, with every member of the community seeking God. At the same time, his Rule is grounded in daily reality. Benedict addresses areas as simple as the tools of the monastery, clothing, food, and how to treat guests. The Rule, as Benedictine sister and author Joan Chittister explains, "simply takes the dust and clay of every day and turns it into beauty."[1]

While we don't know a great deal about Benedict, we do know that he was born around 480 C.E. to a fairly well-to-do family. He lived in Nursia in Italy, during a time of intense upheaval in Europe. Rome itself had been invaded in 410 C.E. by tribes from the north of Europe. Much that had been known and trusted within his society had been destroyed by ongoing warfare. Benedict studied in Rome, but became disillusioned by the behavior he saw in the city, so he dropped out of school and left the city. From there he went eventually to Subiaco, where he began to live as a hermit in a cave. As word of his devotion spread, others came to be with him. As that community grew, he founded twelve small monasteries in the surrounding area, communities that needed some structured way of living together. His first attempt at drafting a rule of life for the community provoked rebellion; his followers turned on him and even sought to poison him! Benedict left Subiaco for Monte Cassino, where it is believed that he wrote the Rule as we know it. He drew on other rules that were already known, creating a pattern for communal life that emphasized balance and moderation.

The Rule of St. Benedict is full of homely and practical wisdom. Joan Chittister has commented, "If we are not spiritual where we are and as we are, we are not spiritual at all."[2] Benedict's way of living is grounded in reality, in daily life, in care of the body and respect for one another, in the intersection of the commandments to love God and love our neighbor as ourselves. As we begin to reflect on living with illness as a rule of life, Benedict's counsel offers some direction and humane encouragement.

My own rule, before my illness, revolved around myriad activities and varied interests. I prayed and read scripture daily. I tried to live a reflective life that noticed God's presence in the daily minutiae of life with teenage sons, work as a parish priest, marriage to a priest. I was finding new avenues for outreach ministry, interviewing clients at an ecumenical hunger ministry, and becoming involved in interfaith dialogue. Gardening and yoga were also part of my rule. Those simple patterns for putting God at the center were very important to me. And they were completely disrupted and torn apart by the illness and the terrible, slow recovery. I had to begin again and find a new way of ordering my life. I had to take into account a severely weakened physical condition. A whole host of new behaviors needed to be practiced—everything from regular rest to meal planning to having blood tests. Slowly, over the months of waiting for healing, a new rule began to emerge. This was a rule that began with the restrictions caused by the illness. This was a rule whose parameters were determined by a life lived within new limitations, limitations that made me want to rebel, to cry, to give up. Surprisingly, those same limitations became the raw material from which a rule could emerge, once I was guided to see them from a different perspective. I started to apply some creativity and prayer to the enterprise of reshaping my new life.

As I did this I realized that *the illness itself provided the grounding for the new rule.* My body, now foreign territory to me in its thoroughly depleted condition, offered the place from which the new rule could grow. Very slowly, I began to see that the rest that the doctor recommended could be one piece of the new rule. The highly restricted diet could be another. Regular ingestion of prescribed medications—something that was tremendously difficult for me in the beginning—became a kind of prayer of the hours. Taking those medications several times daily required a sort of concentration and attention that seemed almost like listening prayer. The rhythm of a day punctuated by times of taking pills was oddly reminiscent of a day marked by praying Morning Prayer, Noonday Prayer, Evening Prayer, and Compline. The living God who is with us in all circumstances and through all passages began to be surprisingly present in these altered patterns of daily life. So, the rudiments of a new rule of life began to appear in the midst of the wreckage of a life shattered by acute illness. Those rudiments were found in the living *with* the illness, in the daily recognition of myself as one weakened and afflicted, yet also upheld and sustained by God.

Beginning Again, Again

The illness forced me to rethink my daily routines and how I live my life. I had to begin again. Since the original attack in 1995, I have had to begin again several times. The fall of 2002 was plagued by sudden flare-ups of pain and concluded with a procedure to open up a restricted duct that was clogged by scar tissue. Most of the plans I'd made for those months were discarded. The recurring bouts of pancreatic disturbance took precedence over any plans, and everything else had to be rearranged. Beginning again, yet again.

Living with illness is definitely full of surprises, punctuated, sometimes, by setbacks. It is also an ongoing lesson in flexibility, resilience, and perseverance. From the vantage point of my mid-fifties, it seems to me that living with illness offers an intensive course in the rule of life. Illness clarifies what really matters, what is worth spending time on, what is essential. Mid-life offers that course to almost everyone over forty; living with illness focuses and concentrates that instruction. In some ways living with illness reminds me of taking an intensive Italian class in college. Class met every day, and only by showing up for class could we learn the language. Living with illness puts you into the same kind of intensive learning situation. When you "show up" by paying attention and becoming more aware of the shape of your life with illness, you begin to learn the new "language."

At this point in my life, I live with a pancreas that has healed to a certain extent. I am still taking medication, still following a particular dietary regimen, and am still afflicted from time to time by pancreatic pain. I have also been working with some groups of people who live with illness. Several years ago in a class I taught at St. Mark's, my Episcopal parish in San Antonio, I suggested that we begin to look at the limitations and diminishments of illness as the beginnings of a new rule of life. At first, the participants were jarred by the idea. How could illness be a rule of *life*? How could these various indignities and limitations have anything to do with vitality, with liveliness, with choosing life? How could God be at the center of living with the diminishments of illness?

Together we began to "re-frame" living with illness. We named our various limitations. We listed the "givens" that each of us

lived with. These varied from person to person, from illness to illness. The person whose diabetes required regular insulin injections and checks of blood sugar had different limitations than the
person whose five years of coexistence with a lymphoma had
resulted in yet another experimental protocol of chemotherapy.
Each "given" traced the outline of life with a particular illness. For
example, the dietary routine of an insulin-dependent diabetic
gave her the frame from which her rule began. The man recovering from a stroke discovered that his regular physical therapy was
the foundation for his rule. These "givens" that come from living
with the illness were the building blocks for a rule of life. Each
"given" also proved to be the starting point for reflecting anew,
for finding a rule of life in the midst of the ongoing rounds of
tests, exams, hospitalizations.

After the class had met for several weeks, one participant
remarked, "This is beginning to give all this mess some meaning."
Redefining the illness led to looking for ways to choose life in the
midst of daily physical distress. We were not trying to deny the
fact of illness, nor to paint the experience with Pollyanna-pink
tones. But we learned that even within the "givens" of living with
illness, there was a lot of rich variety. One woman confined to a
wheelchair said, "When I started paying attention, I realized that
people talk to me now about their own difficulties. I don't necessarily go looking for them. They see me and I'm not so threaten-
ing. I'm less lonely now than I was as a healthy person." A man
with a progressive illness realized that the illness had helped him
see the extent to which his work had become a very controlling
idol. As he let go of the demands of work because of the greater
demands of his body, he realized the illness had been a kind of
salvation. It led him to let go of work as an idol and helped him
examine other values he held in his life.

If you are living with illness, this book offers some suggestions
for transforming the way you perceive the limits that your illness

may place on you. While acknowledging the hard losses that many face when illness overtakes their lives, this text is also written with the conviction that living with illness offers an opportunity to begin anew. That does not mean it is easy. Nor does it mean that living with illness is a happy experience. It does mean that out of the wreckage, piece by piece, with companions along the way, we can begin to discern life that is rich, vital, and real. It may not look at all like the life that we lost. Yet it does have its own singular meaning and character—even beauty—if we allow ourselves the time and patience for discovery.

In the first part of this book, I will reflect on the pattern of dying and rising to new life that is the pattern of Christian baptismal life. In the chapters that follow I invite you to join me in reflecting on a variety of aspects of living with illness—nutrition, rest, exercise, medications, treatment. If one of these chapters doesn't apply to you, feel free to skip it. Choose what is appropriate for your own life, for your particular illness (or, if you are a caregiver, for your own life with this person who is suffering from illness).

In the third section we will look at the three vows of the Rule of St. Benedict: stability, obedience, and ongoing conversion. These chapters offer suggestions about the ways that the vows monks and nuns take might apply to living with your illness. Each chapter ends with suggestions for reflection and with a short prayer. If you intend to follow the suggestions for reflection, I would recommend that you have a journal at hand. Any kind of journal—from a spiral notebook to a fancy blank book—will work fine. Those of you who decide to try some of the suggestions that include an artistic response will want to have crayons or colored markers and some blank paper at hand. I prefer to use a spiral-bound sketchbook with blank pages that allows my writing and art to be in the same journal.

As with any aspect of the journey of faith, it is good and essential to have companions along the way. As you read this book, you will discover that there are suggestions for reflection, prayer, and practice. All of these are simply suggestions. I invite you to include your spiritual companions in this journey, so that they may pray for you as you go along. You may from time to time decide that something has come up that you need to take to a spiritual director or discuss with your physician. My hope is that each reader will invite appropriate friends and professionals into the ongoing process of discerning how to live faithfully with illness.

In these pages you will find a way to discover the rule of life that your own experience of illness offers—a rule that is grounded in the reality of the nutrition, rest, medications, and treatment that are part of your life and needs. Throughout the book, you will find stories from others who have lived with illness and have found ways to discover God's presence in the midst of their daily struggles. The names of these people have been changed, and their stories are used with permission.

Let us begin again.

2

Discerning Your Rule of Life:
Learning to Listen

In 1996, I ended up in the hospital again. Because my white cell count was habitually low, I had to have a bone marrow biopsy. When the hematologist came into the room to perform the procedure, I asked if he thought this was really necessary. "At the very least, it will allow your doctor to rule out a lot of things," he replied. "Then she can start anew from there."

Living with illness rules out a lot of things. Those of you who have illness as a daily companion know all about this. Yet the loss of some things in your life also opens up space for unexpected beginnings. Those beginnings may seem small and very vulnerable, as all brand new life is, yet those beginnings tell us that in the midst of the illness, renewal is occurring.

There is a saying from the Japanese Zen tradition: "Now that my house has burned down I own a better view of the moon" (Masahide). Our bodily houses may have "burned down," but seen another way, we are now invited to notice not only what has been consumed, but what may be present in beautiful simplicity, like the full moon on a windswept night. We can begin to see things we missed before. "Always we begin again,"[1] wrote Benedict in his Rule. Our "burned down house" invites us to begin again, to develop a new rule of life that acknowledges that our life has changed.

Developing or revising your rule of life may seem like a daunting project, but it doesn't need to be that way. Start with just observing your life. As you begin again, try to know your life as your life *with*, rather than *against* or *in spite of*, your illness. Each day brings reminders of what has been lost, but try to notice what is present as well. You are invited to remember the life that you had, and you are invited to bless the life you are being given, in whatever limited form that may be.

When we live with illness and let it help us establish a new rule of life, we act in faith. We acknowledge the astounding possibility that God will be with us in every frightening and distressing moment of the illness. We learn to expect glimpses of divine presence in the most absurd circumstances—from being sick following chemotherapy to being punctured and probed in medical tests. Living with a rule of life helps us to undo what is false or no longer pertinent. Work on establishing a rule that is grounded in present reality, that is based on what *is*, rather than what *could have been*. As a spiritual director once told me, "Begin where you are, not where you are not." Once illness has become an integral part of your life, there may be a temptation to live an illusion— to live as if your body does not need extra care, as if you are capable of the workload you previously carried, as if the illness has made no difference. Even when an illness is fairly manageable, its very presence confronts us with that most basic and most avoided human reality: we are mortal and one day we will die. Very little in our culture helps us to live, as the Rule of St. Benedict counsels, remembering daily that we will die.[2] Illness, for better or for worse, helps us live more consciously. The awareness of our mortality may actually become the gift of experiencing life more deeply while we walk on this earth.

Listening with the Ear of the Heart

The first line of the Prologue to the Rule of St. Benedict reads, "Listen carefully, my child, to my instructions, and attend to them with the ear of your heart."[3] In *Broken Body, Healing Spirit: Lectio Divina and Living with Illness*, I suggested that Benedict invites us to listen to our bodies and to our lives. Living with illness always changes our lives. Normal routine is disrupted. Habits of exercise, travel, work, and play may have to be reconfigured. Though some of the changes that we need to make may be obvious or dictated, discerning some part of our new rule of life requires that we listen deeply to our own experiences of living with illness.

But how do we begin to listen to the body that is stricken with illness, to listen to the altered pattern, to listen to the unspoken grief and sadness and pain? We begin by taking the time to reflect, to remember, to recollect. We need to stop or slow down long enough to reflect on what has happened, what we are observing about ourselves and the new world, and what our responses to all of it are. But that kind of listening to our lives may make us uncomfortable, particularly when illness is involved. If we are honest, if we name the realities of our new life with illness to and for ourselves, we may stir up all sorts of feelings and fears that we would prefer to ignore.

In this respect, a rule that begins with listening leads us into deeper truth. Listening with the ear of the heart to God and for God in the ragged details of our lives invites us to be realistic, to be mindful of our limitations, and to welcome a deepening gratitude. In this quiet listening, you will hear your soul speak, and you will begin to recognize the genuine expression of your life within the limits of illness.

In his book *Let Your Life Speak*, Quaker author Parker Palmer notes, "Verbalizing is not the only way our lives speak, of course.

They speak through our actions and reactions, our intuitions and instincts, our feelings and bodily states of being, perhaps more profoundly than through our words. We are like plants, full of tropisms that draw us toward certain experiences and repel us from others. If we can learn to read our own responses to our own experience—a text we are writing unconsciously every day we spend on earth—we will receive the guidance we need to live more authentic lives."[4] So it is that in listening to our bodies, to the routines imposed by illness, to the contexts in which the illness places us, we begin to hear our own life and to discern its new and different rhythms.

Joan Chittister has observed, "The spiritual life is achieved only by listening to all of life and learning to respond to each of its dimensions wholly and with integrity."[5] When you listen to the changes that come about because of illness, you may indeed encounter sadness or sorrow or discomfort, or even anger or fear. But you may also discover real thankfulness, a sudden awareness of the fragility of life, and a renewed clarity of the unique value of all created things.

Listening to and for God in the midst of loss is in itself an act of trust. Oftentimes illness forces us to think more clearly about God and even to renegotiate our relationship with God. You might, for instance, uncover an assumption that God has abandoned you, or, worse yet, that God has somehow been the cause of your illness. You may discover that you have unconsciously assumed that God has a mean streak and chooses to sic illness on those who misbehave. Once you realize that kind of assumption is operating within you, without your recognizing it, you can deal with the assumption and throw out the image, and look for the living God to be revealed even in the valley of the shadow of death. In my own practice of this kind of listening, I have discovered some old images of God that were buried in my psyche. Patient work with my spiritual director helped me see God in new ways: God eternally with each of us, within our very cells, hallowing our sufferings by abiding with us and walking with us every second. The divine presence also has broken through for me in tender, maternal ways, embodied in the kindness of nurses and physicians, in the ministrations of nurses aides and lab technicians. Some suggestions for developing the habit of listening to your life and to God within it follow.

Suggestions for Reflection

1. What kinds of losses have you experienced because of the illness? These might include loss of mobility, of health, of the way in which you perceived yourself, of faith. Begin to write these losses down, updating your list as things occur to you. Be as specific as you can. What feelings do you have about these losses? Bring them to God in prayer. For example, once you have made your initial list, read each entry out loud and pray, "Into your hand I commit my spirit; you have redeemed me, O Lord, faithful God" (Psalm 31:5).

2. What signs of new life have you begun to note? New life might include slowly returning strength or glimmers of altered identity. Maybe you've made new friends in the doctor's waiting room or during chemotherapy treatments. Perhaps the first new hairs are appearing on your head after chemotherapy. Or you might have just learned to stand again after a long time of weakness. If you are not yet able to see new life within the illness, be honest about that. Let yourself tell the truth. If you are seeing some evidence of returning health, some intimation of physical stability, or other signs of new life, offer prayers of thanksgiving. I sometimes pray after each listing, "You are the God who works wonders; I bless You for blessing me."

3. As you reflect on signs of new life, you might want to try to depict this with color instead of, or in addition to, your words. In your journal or on a blank piece of paper, simply draw or paint "new life." Crayons or colored markers work well for this practice. Jill, who wanted to celebrate the removal of sutures following a cancer surgery, drew a simple outline of her body, the line of the scar from the incision, and multicolored flowers growing from the scar. She said it felt like the flowering of the cross at Easter. Tom drew a heart in red and pink after his heart bypass. Though his body still hurt from the procedure, the drawing gave him a sense of the healing that was happening beyond his sight. This is not an exercise in artistry. This is a way to listen to your life, to give your soul a chance to speak, to pray with color. Once you have finished, you may want to put the color rendition of "new life" in a place where you can see it daily and use it as a springboard for prayer.

4. In her book *Living Faith Day by Day*, author Debra Farrington suggests that we begin to formulate a rule of life by making a list of what feeds our spirits.[6] Begin such a list for yourself. If you are in a severely weakened state, what feeds your spirit may be something as gentle as watching the finches at the birdfeeder, or listening to music you love. Even if your body is weakened, you will still have ways to feed your spirit. These may not be the same things that used to feed you before the illness began, but there will still be sights, sounds, or activities that quicken and nurture your spirit, even in the midst of illness.

The responses to these four questions are the basic material from which your rule will grow as you progress through this book.

From time to time, you will want to return to these questions, reconsider them, add to or change what you've written.

Prayer

Almighty and everlasting God, the comfort of the sad and the strength of those who suffer, hear the prayers of your people who are in any trouble. Grant to everyone in distress mercy, relief, and refreshment; through Jesus Christ our Lord. Amen.[7]

3

Dying and Rising

Kitty lived for over twenty years with breast cancer. Diagnosed initially when she was a young mother with two daughters of elementary school age, Kitty survived five different recurrences of her cancer. She underwent many different protocols, some of them experimental. She lived through many seasons of dying and rising. She had the sense to recognize that the cancer brought her an uncommon awareness—she knew from her thirties that she could, as the poet Naomi Shihab Nye puts it, "tumble any second." Kitty had lived long enough to see each of her daughters married and to be present for the birth of her grandchildren. Over the years of treatments and surgeries, she developed a rule—a way of living—that focused on the present moment. She allowed herself the luxury of being with those whom she loved, of celebrating family holidays with great joy and silliness, of indulging in some of the ways in which her spirit was fed. In all of this, when a recurrence happened, she went again through a kind of dying. What she had known had fallen away. Different treatment regimens required new strategies, and Kitty regularly had to readjust patterns of eating, sleeping, and exercise in response to a recurrence and its treatment. On occasion she lived with a sense of emptiness for months. Then, something new would begin to make itself known.

When Kitty finally came to the end of her earthly life, she was well prepared for a holy dying. Though every person who knew and loved her hoped for even more years of life for her, it was clear that she was ready, that her practice of tending to the pattern of dying and rising had given her a way to negotiate her final days. Her sense of humor remained intact to the end, as well as some of her slightly eccentric behavior.

Over the twenty years of living with cancer, Kitty was honest with herself, her husband, her family, and her clergy about the sadness, the fear, the pain, the sometimes interminable weakness. At the same time, Kitty welcomed the rising to new life when it came. She reached out to other women living with breast cancer, sharing generously what she had learned, from coping strategies to the names of oncologists. Knowing she could tumble any second, she had decided what to do with her time.

At the heart of all human life, whether we are aware of it or not, is the pattern of dying and rising. Each night when we go to sleep, we experience an ending, a little death. The day we have just lived is gone forever. Each morning when we rise, we rise a slightly different person than we were the morning before. The previous day's conversations, encounters, circumstances, and relationships have altered us just a little.

We also die and rise on an annual cycle. As I write these words, autumn is coming to central Texas. The sky changes radically as the north winds blow the moisture from the Gulf of Mexico back to its origin. The light shifts. Flocks of geese and ducks are occasionally sighted, even from city streets, as the primal stirrings lead them toward their autumnal migrations. The earth prepares for the dying off of each spring's growth, each summer's harvest. As the air cools and the leaves cascade to the earth, we find ourselves directed inwardly, recognizing that the beauty of the fall colors signals the prelude to winter. In her poem "The Art of Disappearing," the poet Naomi Shihab Nye counsels:

> *Walk around feeling like a leaf.*
> *Knowing you could tumble any second*
> Then *decide what to do with your time.*[1]

There is a profound wisdom in this kind of awareness, the kind that remembers both the fragility and the resilience of all life.

The longer we live, the more we recognize that winter is always followed by spring. In the deep stillness of winter, we are brought into a kind of unknowing that is a mercy. There is a mercy in discovering that we are not the source of our own life. There is a mercy in recognizing the divine power that continually brings life out of death. We come up against the limits of our own knowledge and experience. We "unknow" ourselves as being the sole authors of our existence. This unknowing delivers us from our assumptions, our arrogance, our silly notions that we are in control of our lives, of our selves, of our bodies. When spring stirs, we are often surprised. The garden that existed in our imaginations has its own life and its own mystery. Seeds that we'd forgotten we planted begin to sprout. Other seeds sprout, but never come to full growth.

Two years ago I planted hollyhock seeds given to me by a friend. No sooner had I planted them than central Texas was inundated with torrential rain. No hollyhock sprouts appeared. I assumed the seeds had either been completely swept away in the fifteen inches of rain, or that they had drowned.

Last spring, an odd-looking shoot appeared in my herb garden. As it began to grow, to unfold its first leaves, to gain stature and strength, I realized with a jolt that it was a hollyhock. The plant grew to an astounding seven feet and was literally a mass of hot pink blossoms. In my own backyard, the pattern of dying and rising startled me into paying attention. In its own time—rather than mine—this one seed germinated. When I thought there was no possibility of a hollyhock, much less one of such abundance and strength, it appeared, offering pink blossoms worthy of the brush of Georgia O'Keefe.

Dying and rising happens continually in our bodies. Medical science tells us that on the cellular level we are continually being made new. Old cells die off. New cells are brought into being. Our physical selves, our bodies, through all of the mysterious trans-formational processes of respiration, digestion, elimination, are silently, quietly living out the pattern of dying and rising—even when we are in the best of health. And when we are living with an illness, even when that illness is the dominant shaping force in our lives, the cellular dying and rising still happens. This happens through an agency that is not our own. We can support this process. We can impede it. We do not, however, cause it to happen. This flesh that we so often denigrate and despise, particularly when it is no longer functioning at what we perceive to be an optimal level, continues to be the space "wherein the Holy Spirit makes a dwelling."[2] The Holy Spirit who has knit us together in our mother's wombs continues to knit together new cells, new tissue, new flesh.

Those of us who are members of the Christian faith tradition are explicitly, sacramentally participants in a pattern of dying and rising by virtue of our baptisms. In my own tradition, that of the Episcopal Church, we understand, as Saint Paul did, that we are baptized into Christ's death and resurrection. As the water for baptism is blessed, we pray: "We thank you, Father, for the water of Baptism. In it we are buried with Christ in his death. By it we share in his resurrection. Through it we are reborn by the Holy Spirit."[3]

Baptism marks the beginning of our preparation for a holy dying and a holy rising. This is to be a daily pattern, an integration of allowing what needs to die in us to do so, and making space for what Christ is calling forth through the power of his resurrection. Here is the deepest mystery of our faith: that in our losses, in our sufferings, in our pains, in our dying, God in Christ is with us. Furthermore, through the power of that Holy Spirit that moves within us in sighs too deep for words, new life is possible. The Spirit, the Giver of Life as the Nicene Creed proclaims, gives life when we least expect it. The same Spirit that moved over the waters of creation, moves over us and in us. New life is possible even when the body is failing, even in the throes of terminal illness. As we say in the burial service: "Even at the grave we make our song: Alleluia, alleluia, alleluia."[4]

Living with a rule of life is a way of tending to the patterns of dying and rising. A rule invites us to notice what we need to let go of. It helps us to notice areas of our lives that are begging for mercy, for new orientation, for the quickening soft breath of God's own spirit, for repentance. As we seek to recognize God at the center of all that we are and all that we have, our priorities will change. And even small changes in our priorities can rearrange the entire design of our lives. It is sort of like a kaleidoscope—a small turn of the lens results in a completely new pattern.

Illness often turns that lens whether we want it turned or not. It may take months or even years for us to accept the turning of that lens that a diagnosis of chronic or progressive illness presents. Several seasons may pass before we can discern any beauty or color in the pattern that the illness brings into being.

The Benedictine Rule counsels, "Always we begin again." Always a rising follows the dying. Ours is a God who calls forth life from death. Ours is a God who brings forth life in ways we never expected, in circumstances in which new life never seemed possible. Our first invitation is to recognize the dying, to name it, to hallow it, to bring it to speech. We need to notice that the lens of the kaleidoscope of our lives has indeed been turned, that our life has been altered, in many cases, for the rest of our earthly days.

We recognize the dying of our life as we know it by squarely facing the empty tomb. The empty tomb always startles us. Death creates an empty space. In that pause, that moment of emptiness, before the rising has been sighted, we are jolted out of old perceptions. The frame of reality shifts. The physical limitations forced on us by chronic illness often feel like a kind of dying. We find ourselves, as Jesus did for a period, among the dead—among the deadness in ourselves and in our flesh. We feel out of control. We're in territory we don't recognize or understand. This is a time of unknowing.

As we adjust to the fact of illness, to its ever-present reality in our lives, we may need to grieve. We may need to name the losses we've experienced as a result of living with illness. One person needs to grieve the loss of physical mobility. Others grieve lost parts of their bodies. Still others may be trying to come to terms with vastly diminished days of this life.

One of my favorite prayers from The Book of Common Prayer contains this line: "Make us, we pray, deeply aware of the shortness and uncertainty of human life."[5] When you stop and think about it, that's a pretty strange prayer. Most of us don't like to be reminded how easily a life can end. But living with illness can force us to face the shortness and uncertainty of human life, like it or not. We know in our bones that we could, like the autumn leaf, fall at any moment, and naming that and experiencing our feelings around that awareness are essential.

In the Christian tradition, the faithful are encouraged to prepare for a holy dying. Christians are encouraged to face death in humility, aware of the gracious gift of life, prepared to be received into the arms of God's mercy, into the blessed rest of everlasting peace, and into the glorious company of the saints in light.[6] When we practice the hallowing of our little dyings, we are learning what a holy death might look like. When we recognize a dying that comes with living with illness—whether that dying is the loss of a particular self-image, the need to change employment, the inability to participate in a favorite pastime or sport—we can bring the dying to prayer. We can speak aloud our sadness over the loss, and we may be softened by the gift of tears. We also may uncover real anger over the loss. Perhaps we will discover residual bitterness or resentment.

In noticing the dyings, in naming them and being open to the feelings from which we may have hidden, we make room for new life to come. We allow resurrection to happen. We enter that moment of deepest trust, that moment when we hope for signs of new life, even when we see no evidence of it. We wait in hope. We participate in the promise that is in creation itself—in the turning of night to day, in the giving way of winter frost to spring's stirrings, in the continual dying and remaking of cells in our bodies. We hang on to and live out the promise of Christian baptism and the proclamation of Easter that we will be granted new life. That new life usually comes in a form we did not anticipate, and perhaps in a way we would never have wished. Yet the life comes nonetheless.

Suggestions for Reflection

1. In your own experience of living with illness, reflect on the patterns of dying and rising that you have come to know. In what ways has your illness taught you about loss? What specific griefs have you lived with since your initial diagnosis and treatment? As you write these down, notice the feelings that arise. There may be residual sadness, or anger, or resentment. There may be a kind of tender wistfulness over dreams that will never come to pass. Let

yourself write what you need to write. If writing is not possible for you, you might try using a tape recorder and just speaking your thoughts aloud.

Once your list is made (you may want to refer back to your answers at the end of chapter 2) pray each loss. Name the loss, using the formula, "I name before God the loss of. . . ." Then respond to the naming with, "Into your hands O Lord, I commend my former life." This will create a kind of a litany, a prayer with a regular response. Here's a sample of what this might look like:

"I name before God the loss of my health."
"Into your hands, O Lord, I commend my former life."
"I name before God the loss of my stamina."
"Into your hands, O Lord, I commend my former life."
"I name before God the loss of my ability to run."
"Into your hands, O Lord, I commend my former life."

Prayerfully, gently, acknowledge what you need to let go.

If you choose, use the crayons or markers to draw some of these losses. This could be as simple as one color on a sheet of paper, bringing your prayer into form. If handling art supplies is too difficult, you could gently meditate on each named loss, simply pausing after each naming and letting yourself become aware of the feelings and bodily responses to the loss.

This particular exercise is one that may also be done in the wise presence of a spiritual friend or companion or director. Simply allowing yourself to name these dyings in the presence of another trusted person shares the sadness and invites the small beginnings of transformation. A gifted listener helps us hear what we are saying, what we might otherwise miss. For example, one wise older friend of mine caught my use of a particular phrase that seemed to signal that on some level I was aware of the healing. Until she saw those little clues of new life in my speech and pointed them out to me, I was unaware of the subtle shift that was already occurring.

2. How are you beginning to decide what to do with your time? In what ways has the illness helped you in this process of discernment?

3. Reflect on how your daily pattern has changed as a result of living with illness. What marks your days? How are your daily needs for sleep, nutrition, medication, exercise, prayer, and community lived out? How is this different from your pre-illness life? How is it similar?

4. Do you have a sense that your illness has been a teacher? Have you gleaned any wisdom because of living with an illness? What have you learned? Make note of this, and give thanks.

5. As you reflect on ways in which the pattern of dying and rising has been manifest in your life, are you aware of ways in which the illness has helped you become more yourself? Some people discover that an illness has the potential to deliver them from unnoticed habits that were not helpful or healthy. Note any ways in which your experience of living with illness has allowed you to listen to your deep life.

Prayer

I believe, O Lord and God of the peoples,
That Thou art He Who created my soul and set its warp,
Who created my body from dust and from ashes,
Who gave to my body breath, and to my soul its possessions.
Father, bless to me my body,
Father, bless to me my soul,
Father, bless to me my life,
Father, bless to me my belief.[7]

PART II

LIVING WITH ILLNESS:
DISCOVERING YOUR RULE OF LIFE

4

Nutrition and Mindful Eating

I n 1995, when I first came home from the hospital after the attack of acute pancreatitis, I could hardly eat anything. Runny oatmeal was the best I could manage, along with Popsicles™ and Jell-O™. Anything more challenging than clear broth with a little rice and chicken produced cold sweats and pain. Before the attack I had already been following a low-fat diet, having discovered, several months earlier, that my cholesterol levels were elevated. That was an adjustment in and of itself. I was brought up loving both the chicken-fried steak and mashed potato meals of Texas, and the cheese enchilada with *chile con carne* feasts of Tex-Mex "regular plates" from favorite restaurants. Now, the foods I could readily digest were few. I was in a survival mode. In other words, if I were to survive, if I were to allow my damaged body to heal, I would have to eat very differently.

In some ways, those long months in 1995 and 1996 were like an extended fast. I am on a permanent fast from alcohol, from fatty foods, from anything fried. In my case, deviation from the fast produces sharp pain, not just the slow sludging of arteries. The pancreas, delicate and mysterious organ that it is, tends to pitch a fit when any of these foods are introduced to the digestive tract. My body insists on the fast, not just for today or for this week but for the rest of my life.

Any of you who live with an illness that requires steady attention to nutrition and patterns of eating have probably discovered the same kind of limitation. If you live with diabetes, you may find yourself weighing your food and needing to balance food groups as you plan meals for a day. Those of you on kidney dialysis are trying to cope with a lengthy list of foods that you're not allowed to eat. Others who live with food allergies, sometimes life-threatening ones, also spend time carefully reading labels in the grocery store and ordering meals in restaurants with attention to detail.

All of these necessary practices invite us to make nutrition and mindful eating part of our rule of life. In my own experience, having to pay such close attention to the basic need to eat has made me acutely aware of many layers of dependence and interdependence. For example, I initially had to eat many small meals, like babies do. The foods I could eat were often the consistency of baby food. Though I was feeding myself, it was impossible for me to avoid the message: if I were going to live with this ailment, I would need to take care of myself as I cared for my own sons in their infancy. At first this felt downright embarrassing, even though I could hardly get out of bed. How could a formerly self-sufficient (hah!), energetic professional woman deal with having to feed herself as if she were a toddler?

Gradually I came to realize that this kind of feeding puts God in the center of nourishing the body. I think of this as a kind of co-creating, of working with God by supporting and appropriately feeding vulnerable new life. This kind of feeding takes you back to basics. Our bodies need food in order to live. When we are newborn, we can't manage spaghetti and meatballs. When we are beginning again, we need the right food for that beginning. Feeding myself was, first and foremost, the practical and necessary action for supplying enough energy to live through the day. If we don't eat, eventually we die. If we don't eat appropriately, eventually our bodies suffer ill effects.

In his Rule, Benedict made provision for the feeding of the community, while also being mindful of the needs of the young, the elderly, the ill. He was concerned that the members of the community received the proper amount of food, and that at each table two kinds of cooked food were available. "In this way," Benedict wrote, "the person who may not be able to eat one kind of food may partake of the other. Two kinds of cooked food, therefore should suffice for all the brothers, and if fruit or fresh vegetables are available, a third dish may be added."[1] Benedict also stipulated the providing of a pound of bread per day. He takes care to note that heavy labor may require heartier food, though meat from four-footed animals is not permitted. For those who are ill, meat is allowed so that they may regain their strength.

Benedict recognized that within each community each monk may have particular needs. He provided for those needs. He also provided for the changing of seasons with regard to the times of meals. Benedict demonstrates a keen awareness of the natural rhythms of the seasons. Mindful of the cost of manual labor in summer heat, Benedict allows that the abbot should arrange all matters "that souls may be saved and the brothers may go about their activities without justifiable grumbling."[2] Benedict's counsel with regard to food and rhythm helped me to approach my own nourishment with a gentler attitude. The bald necessity of careful, attentive eating pushed aside much that had formerly taken my attention—books, theological wrangling, pastoral concern, politics. Now I was trying to plan something to feed myself every two to three hours. I was trying to get sufficient calories and vitamins into my food, without provoking a pancreatic disturbance.

If you have ever lived through similar circumstances, you know that this focus on eating leads us to reflect on the contingency of our lives. I felt very vulnerable, and I felt sad. I didn't want to begin again in this way. I didn't want to watch my body waste away daily. Looking in the mirror became difficult. Many of you who have endured cancer know a similar kind of sadness in watching your body deteriorate from treatment and disease.

Nutrition became an essential aspect of my ongoing rule of life. Even though I am relatively stable at present, I still need to be very attentive to what I eat. If I go to a restaurant, 75–80 percent of what is on the menu is not food I should put in my mouth— not because it is bad food, but because it is not the right food for me. If I go to a diocesan meeting at which lunch is to be served, I have learned it is wise to pack my own food, because often something that I absolutely cannot have is served.

What Is the Food that Is Good for You?

This growing clarity that not all good food is good for me became another piece of the nutritional component of my own rule of life. Realizing this also taught me to prioritize other kinds of "food," other things that were supposed to nurture me, such as what I read, what I listen to, what I watch. We ingest all of these, just as we ingest food, and they become part of our reality. The nutritional demands of the pancreatic condition led me to reflect on "nutrition" in my life as a whole. I started paying more attention to what I was "feeding" myself in terms of watching television or listening to the radio. I began to notice that I no longer had such an omnivorous appetite, desiring to learn anything new or thought-provoking, wanting to gobble up all kinds of experience. I started discovering what I *really* desired to "eat," to take in, to feed upon.

Inevitably, this became connected to receiving the sacrament of the Body of Christ by participating in Holy Communion. I began to regard the nutritional part of this rule as an ongoing discernment of what truly constituted the bread of life. To push the metaphor a bit, I didn't want to eat mass-produced white sandwich bread with no food value. It was a waste of calories and a waste of digestive energy. I wanted to be receiving bread full of life, bread that would, in turn, give me life. The spiritual and metaphorical ramifications of this piece of my nutritional rule of life continue to unfold, sometimes when I least expect it.

In a class I led on living with illness as a rule of life, several of the class members discovered that in learning to feed themselves well and in a way appropriate to the demands of the illness, they could be amazingly creative. They began to discover creative ways to prepare food. But they also discovered that they could be creative with how the food was placed on the plate, the kitchen environment, the dining area, and setting the table. In other words, each meal had the potential for becoming Holy Communion.

One participant said, "You know, I keep thinking about the fact that I did not grow this food. I realize that the food comes to me through the labor of others." As we reflected together, we began to recognize that tending this part of the rule led us not only to awareness about how and what we feed ourselves, but to a deepening gratitude for the unknown persons who raised the vegetables and fruits, baked the bread, caught the fish, harvested the spices. A wondrous sort of gratitude began to be articulated.

In another instance, a woman in chemotherapy named Diane gave us a tender insight into this deepening sense of connection and communion. Diane had a lifetime practice of eating very little meat, though she did eat fish and poultry. When her treatments seriously depleted her body, her nutritional consultant at the cancer treatment center encouraged her to eat beef liver. The idea was jarring for Diane. Nevertheless, she purchased the prescribed liver at an organic food store. A friend offered to prepare it, as Diane had never cooked liver in her life. The friend took care to place the cooked liver artfully on the plate. In telling me of her experience, Diane remarked, "I swear I could taste the alfalfa that the cow had eaten. I was overwhelmed with gratitude for that creature, for the life she was giving me by the gift of her flesh, for the alfalfa that she'd eaten, for the rancher who had fed her." Deeply moved, Diane tried to find words for this experience, an experience of the communion of all life, revealed in the primal act of feeding herself. She discovered that truth from which we flinch: that our lives are literally fed by the life of other plants and creatures. The sacrifice at the heart of the Eucharist revealed itself in this practice of intentional eating and intentional nutrition.

Suggestions for Reflection

1. What changes to your diet are required by your illness?

2. If you have been living with these changes for some time, what have you noticed about your present nutritional guidelines? For example, if you had to give up fatty foods, do you miss them? Have you felt better without the fatty foods?

3. What prayer practice, if any, have you established with regard to eating and nutrition? If you are not keeping some practice of prayer, begin to create a way to incorporate prayer with nutrition. Begin with simple grace at meals. Allow yourself a moment to become aware of the food as gift. Be mindful of those around the world who are living with your illness who need the proper nutrition and cannot obtain it. Pray for them. Lastly, ask a blessing on those who have grown the fruits and vegetables, raised the grain, caught the fish, and on all who have worked to bring the food to your table. Instead of just keeping a list of foods that are prohibited, make a list of foods that you can eat and that you enjoy. Find ways to celebrate the diversity

of foods that are allowed for your particular nutritional plan. These might include:

a. Finding new recipes that fit your dietary needs. One very good online resource is www.cookinglight.com. There are also many cookbooks for those who live with cancer, heart disease, diabetes, or other illnesses. Your physician may have information on resources for healthy cooking and for nutritional guidelines for your specific illness. Many wellness centers also have staff nutritionists who might be able to guide you in cooking well for your body.

b. Including new herbs in your cooking to add taste and interest to your food. If you have the space, grow herbs in pots so that you have fresh herbs at hand. Even small amounts of fresh herbs can help provide flavor when salt and fats are restricted.

c. Giving thought to the space in which you eat, and choosing to make that space more conducive to dining rather than gobbling. Simple additions to the table or space such as candles or a single flower in a vase can make all the difference. Care in arranging food on the plate can also make your meal more appealing and more like communion.

None of this needs to be costly. It is a matter of attention and care taken in the preparation of the dining area.

5. From time to time, take a moment to imagine the ways in which your food connects you to the larger world. For

example, if you are eating rice, offer thanks for those who grew the plant, for those who harvested the grain, for those who prepared the grain for sale, for those who brought the box or bag of rice to the grocery store, for the grocer who sold it to you. The fact is that our food is a primary way in which we are connected to one another, often throughout the world. Each time we eat, we are participating in a form of communion.

If you wish, try picturing this rather than writing about it. Using your crayons or markers, draw one food that you particularly enjoy, and then picture the connections that come to you as you pray.

Prayer

Bless our hearts
to hear in the breaking of bread
the song of the universe. Amen.[3]

5

Rest

A rule of life that is well crafted helps us to live an ordinary life that is mindful of God's presence. We seek, as Benedictine author Joan Chittister has remarked, "to live the ordinary life extraordinarily well."[1] This becomes more of a challenge when living with illness, particularly in a few key areas. One of those areas is learning to balance rest and activity. Again, the illness itself provides the raw material for a rule that leads us to be grateful for the life we live, despite limitations and losses.

Benedict understood the human rhythms of work, prayer, and rest, and he sought to establish a good balance in the communal life of his monasteries. He did not understand work to be the most important dimension of life. Instead, work was but one aspect of a multi-faceted life shaped by preferring Christ above all else. The Rule provides for individual beds for each monk— an innovation for that time. Clearly good rest allowed each monk to be restored for work and prayer. As we apply Benedictine spirituality to living with illness, the question of balance between rest and activity comes to the fore.

A sudden, unexpected onset of illness often forces rest upon us. Because rest of this sort isn't chosen or even desired you may feel more like rebelling than being grateful. It's natural to feel frustrated by your own inactivity. Fear may even become your companion if you begin to wonder if you will ever return to any degree of regular mobility. A progressive disease such as multiple sclerosis carries with it the potential of diminishing mobility; in these cases resting may seem like giving in to the demands of the illness too soon. But living with illness almost always involves some level of rest, and each person needs to discern what balance of rest and activity will allow the body, mind, and spirit to repair.

Resting can teach us the wisdom of the Jewish practice of *Shabbat*. Abraham Joshua Heschel, Jewish scholar and rabbi, reminds us that the practice of observing *Shabbat*, or Sabbath time, calls us to become aware of the mystery of creation.[2] In the second chapter of Genesis, after the work of creating everything that is, God "rested on the seventh day from all the work that he had done. So God blessed the seventh day and hallowed it, because on it God rested from all the work that he had done in creation" (Genesis 2:2–3). This hallowing of time has divine precedent. It is from the perspective of rest that God beholds what God has spoken into being. We who are in the image and likeness of God are invited to rest, too.

When we regard rest from this perspective, we become more attuned to God's own creative activity within our own bodies— knitting broken bones, authoring and guiding all of the won- drous processes of respiration, digestion, elimination, mending tissues recently severed by surgery. We become aware that we are partners with God in helping our bodies heal as much as they can. We can't, of our own free will and doing, make the process happen, but we can help it along. The practice of Sabbath rest reminds us that we are continually in the hands of the living God; we may dis- cover that this revelation makes us fearful. We may discover that the divine Presence is far more intimate that we had thought. We may recognize the Spirit's movement in our own breathing. Such closeness to the living God may be a bit jarring at first.

Ceasing from our normal, pre-illness patterns gives us an opportunity to discover that we haven't been treating ourselves very graciously. We may come to terms with the fact that our bodies have been laboring for years without much kindness, attention, or gratitude on our part. We may be jolted into the acute awareness—an awareness that is so intrinsic to Jewish theology—that our souls and our bodies are one, and that by unconsciously hurting or pushing our bodies, we have done the same to our souls. It is worth noting that in Hebrew the word *nefesh*, which is often translated as "soul," really connotes the whole person, and is associated with the gullet, with appetite, with desire.

Heschel tells us that the Sabbath rest is a delight to both the soul and the body. "Unless one learns how to relish the taste of Sabbath while still in this world, unless one is initiated in the appreciation of eternal life, one will be unable to enjoy the taste of eternity in the world to come,"[3] writes Heschel. Here is a strange possibility: the imposed rest of illness may be the means by which we begin to savor the taste of eternity in this life. Imposed rest, which at first may feel restrictive and difficult, may be the beginning of perceiving life anew. When you are forced to be still and abstain from frenetic activity, you begin to notice things you hadn't seen before, even though they were right there all along. Even when bed rest is accompanied by feelings of uncomfortable dependency and loss of initiative, there are still opportunities for discerning God close at hand—in breath, in muscles and tendons slowly knitting together after surgery, in the care offered by nurses, family, and friends.

Terry came home thoroughly weakened after several months in an intensive care unit, following a life-threatening experience with pneumonia. He discovered that he needed to rest after simply walking to the bathroom. At first he was both scared and angry—his body lacked stamina and muscular strength. Slowly he began to perceive that in the enforced rest, he could not run away from feelings and thoughts that he had pushed away for years. He had held others at bay, afraid to be vulnerable or open. In the resting, he began to notice both his own hardness, and then the subtle softening of that hardness. He began to intentionally thank each friend who came to his help, each aid who came for physical therapy, each neighbor who brought groceries or delivered mail. The imposed rest also led him over time to practice a regular prayer of thanksgiving. Terry would simply thank God for each person, for what *was* working in his body, for each breath.

Illness may be an occasion for saving your life by losing it (Mark 8:35). So often our deep identity, our true self, is lost in myriad activities and covered over by incessant work. Donna Schaper, a minister and contemporary spirituality writer, has remarked that Sabbath time forces us to look at our attitudes toward work.[4] When Sabbath was forced on me, I discovered I had come perilously close to collapsing my whole identity into who I was at work. As Schaper has observed, this is very dangerous spiritually, for the sense of self is vastly reduced and shrunken. Captive to work identity, we no longer see ourselves from a perspective of faith or prayer or meaning. We discover that we are in a terrible dilemma. In the words of my older son, "The wheel is spinning but the hamster is dead."

For some of you, the rest that is an integral part of the rule of life when living with illness will be a welcome gift. For others, the rest will force a confrontation between notions of what you *should* be doing and what you *can* do. You may stumble into the brick wall of your own resistance to stopping and resting. Some people feel worthless when they're not being productive, as society defines it. Perhaps you will discover that you have no sense of a life outside of work. The rest can feel a little like a wilderness— a place that is disorienting and without boundaries. The Israelites, after leaving Egypt, found the desert disorienting as well. In their trek through unknown territory, God called them to stop being slaves and learn their new identity as the Chosen People. To help them God gave them a pillar of cloud by day and a pillar of fire by night to follow. Sometimes the cloud would stay around for days, and the people would rest until it lifted (Exodus 5–24). Such a process often occurs in living with illness, and one of the real challenges may come in learning to simply rest, to commend yourself into God's hands, and to allow your real feelings, concerns, fears, and hopes to make themselves known to you.

If you feel a sense of rebellion about having to rest, pray through that. Be honest about your own frustration with the lack of strength, the slow healing, the continuing diminishment— whatever frustrates you. Pray as you are, not as you think you should be. If you need to be in bed for most of the day, your prayer could be a request to rest well. If you are so weakened that prayer is impossible right now, let yourself rest in the intercessions of others. Allow yourself to know and to be grateful for the prayers offered for you—often a very humbling experience. We are often not well practiced in the gift of receiving. Resting when living with illness deepens our capacity to be receivers and to recognize the ways in which our lives are interwoven with the lives of others.

Several times this pancreatic condition has forced me to bed for days. As one acupuncturist said to me, "Pancreatitis is a global event for the body." Even when the acute phase recedes from an attack, days of mending follow as the body attempts to return to a healthier state. When the first and worst attack happened in 1995, I spent months resting for most of each day. I didn't have enough energy to do anything else. The attack happened in July. From my bed, over the months of rest that followed, I watched two birdfeeders and some of my garden. I saw summer turn to autumn, and autumn deepen into winter. My cats came and kept me company. Grendel (now of blessed memory) often sat on my

chest as if to say, "Stay put. Rest. Let go." In those months, I sometimes fell prey to depression, particularly to an amorphous sadness. Finally I reached a point of being able to get out of the
house a bit, though I had to be careful about not overdoing. A
friend suggested that I begin to think of "naptime" as a way of
putting a more playful frame on the need to lie down and rest
twice a day. Another friend, who had suffered from a stroke,
handed on advice from her physician: "Befriend your body. Even
if you don't go to sleep, when you rest, you give your wounded
body the chance to recharge, to catch up, to avoid being continually depleted." For some reason, that bit of advice took hold. I
realized that resting was a friendly thing to offer myself, body and
soul. As I thought about "naptime" I remembered that as a child,
I actually liked naps! Someone usually read to me before I went
to sleep, and then they woke me up to some sort of treat like milk
and cookies. As I contemplated my childhood nap experiences, I
realized that there could be a celebratory dimension to the rest.
When I re-read *The Sabbath* by Abraham Joshua Heschel, I saw
that, in part, the imposed rest was leading me to see that I am a
created being, spoken into being by God. Resting began to be a
way to cooperate with the processes of healing, rather than to
work against them. Resting offered me time to reflect, to see, to
remember, to pray. Rest led me to trust that something was happening even if I wasn't the one making it happen. What a surprise!

We need to look to Sabbath time, Heschel notes, as our home-
land, our destination. This is time for independence from social
conditions.[5] As days passed into weeks, and weeks became
months, I realized that some of my real discomfort with inactivity and with resting was giving way to a secret contentment. The
enforced limitations of the illness delivered me from weighty
responsibilities. Some of those responsibilities I cherished and
missed. Others I had begun to have doubts about. It occurred to
me that in this time of enforced rest, I had the opportunity to

cooperate with God's re-creation of my life. The enforced rest helped me understand that whatever my life would look like, it would be very different from what it had been, and that I had a part to play in helping God re-create it. I would not be able to eat anything I wanted to. I would not have the seemingly endless stores of energy that had propelled me through life, allowing me to satisfy enormous curiosity about the world, about the world of spirituality and prayer, about life in general. Instead, I had to choose what to eat, what to do, and to choose well. Following the advice of Joan Chittister, I was learning to choose good from good, and recognizing that this would be a life-long practice.[6]

In the tradition that comes to us from the Desert Fathers and Mothers, we find a saying that helps with this rest dimension of the rule for living with illness. During the fourth century C.E., after Christianity had gained legal status and become an acceptable way of living within all strata of society, many women and men left their cities and began living monastic lives. In silence, stillness, and solitude, they sought to recover something of the rigor and strength of Christian faith lived under threat of persecution. Many of them lived in small huts, or in caves, or in single rooms. "Go to your cell," they were told, "and your cell will teach you everything."

Those who followed the desert tradition had a deep distrust of incessant activity. These women and men understood that ceaseless busyness was one way to create illusions of our own importance, about who we are and what we are here for. Stillness, silence, solitude—that's what they cherished. These were seen as remedies, as means by which a person could seek and be found by God. The monastic cell was both a physical enclosure and a symbol of the heart of the believer. Ultimately, to go to the cell is to go within, to dwell within the silence of one's inner being. Rest during illness is a way of going to your cell. Periods of rest become Sabbath time, a time for being in the eternal regenerative grace of God, even if you are dying. It can also become an opportunity for listening deeply for God's presence. In the night watches, in the resting times during the day, in recovery processes from surgery and medical treatments, you may find that your place of rest becomes a little cell of sorts. Your bed may become a place of prayer. A recliner becomes a prayer closet. A rocker becomes a different kind of "prayer desk."

Ultimately, resting leads many of us to questions of identity. We live in a society in which our identities and our sense of meaning are intimately tied to work, particularly to being "productive." In his fine book *Lifesigns: Intimacy, Fecundity and Ecstasy in Christian Perspective*, author Henri Nouwen observed that we are called to be fruitful, not productive. Productivity emphasizes what we make. We tend, Nouwen observes, to act as if we are what we make.[7] In our culture, we put great emphasis on success and achievement. There is nothing quite like a chronic or progressive illness to put you face to face with this reality and force you to redirect your life away from those ends. Nouwen points us back to the organic nature of bearing fruit, which is what Jesus invites us to do. In the Gospel of John, Jesus says to the disciples, "I am the vine, you are the branches. Those who abide in me and I in them bear much fruit, because apart from me you can do nothing" (John 15:5). Here we have the mystery of mutual indwelling: the living God dwells within us, and we dwell within the living God.

Fruitfulness, or fecundity, is the aim of a faithful life. Nouwen comments, "The great mystery of fecundity is that it becomes visible where we have given up our attempts to control life and take the risk to let life reveal its own inner movements."[8] In being obedient to your ailing body and soul's deep need for rest, you will come to terms with any attempts to control your life. It is hard to exercise control while bedridden, though many people try. When we are in a productive mode, it is easy to live with the illusion that we're doing everything under our own steam, and that we are the ones who make the world. One of the hidden graces of succumbing to the need for ongoing rest is that we discover that when we stop striving, working, and making, the world continues to exist. We begin to realize that there is a life waiting to be lived, a life grounded in hidden organic movement like seeds in the soil. That life will no doubt look very, very different from the life led before becoming ill, but it still has the potential to bear fruit. Just as the seed of an apple can grow into a healthy tree laden with ripe fruit, so, too, can a life plagued by chronic illness be fruitful. The fruit of your life will come from within, sometimes from so deep within that you aren't even aware that there is a seed, much less one that it is sprouting. The fruit will grow forth from your own experience, formed by deepening trust in God and by listening to scripture, to your life, and to wise counsel.

As you go to your cell—whatever that cell is—knowing that your cell will teach you everything, you will soon discover the fruit of being vulnerable. If you can't embrace being vulnerable, pray "I want to be vulnerable about being vulnerable." If you can't stand the fact of your own weakness, pray "I need to be weak enough to say that I am weak." If you hesitate to name your sadness, let that come to speech: "I need to tell You I am sad."

In practicing this sort of vulnerability in prayer, you will begin to practice it with yourself, with your doctors, with your friends, with your family. Vulnerability is a fruit for which we need to acquire a taste. Most of us have very little practice in being appropriately vulnerable. When we do open up a little to God and to one another, relationship that is real and resilient starts to take shape. We don't invest so much energy in keeping the proverbial "stiff upper lip." Honesty, tenderness, and vulnerability go hand in hand—three qualities that are much needed in living with illness.

Honesty begins the nurturing process for whatever seeds await sprouting. Start with gently letting yourself write what you need to write, say what you need to say. In the rest, in the stillness and solitude, you will begin again to hear your deep self speak.

Suggestions for Reflection

1. How does your illness affect the amount of rest you need? Are you able to allow yourself adequate rest? Where do you rest?

2. What is your attitude toward the need to rest? If you are resistant or frustrated by continued weakness, let yourself be honest about that in prayer: "I am tired of being tired." If you are anxious because of your lack of activity, be honest about that. Let yourself explore your feelings about rest.

3. How is your sleep? Are you able to sleep through most of the night or are you wakeful? Sometimes medications interfere with our natural sleep patterns. If you are experiencing a lot of sleep interruption you might want to mention this to your physician. If you find that it happens occasionally, you could regard those wakeful times as opportunity for prayer, especially for intercession for others who are living with your same illness.

4. As you reflect on rest as an essential component of your rule of life, be practical about allowing yourself sufficient rest by avoiding over-scheduling. If your illness permits you to return to work, to resume a somewhat regular daily routine, ask yourself if you are slipping into old habits that are inappropriate to your present life. Notice if you are beginning to force yourself into a "performance mode" that is harmful to the ongoing sustenance of your body.

5. Draw a picture of yourself resting. This does not have to be realistic. It could be a simple line or shape. What colors seem appropriate? Once you have finished the drawing, you might want to write a prayer to go with the drawing. You could use this line from a prayer for the service for Compline: "Give your angels charge over those who sleep."[9]

Prayer

O God of peace, who has taught us that in returning and rest we shall be saved, in quietness and in confidence shall be our strength: By the might of your Spirit lift us, we pray you, to your presence, where we may be still and know that you are God; through Jesus Christ our Lord. Amen.[10]

6
Exercise

For many who live with chronic illness, exercise is an important component of the rule of life. That said, it is imperative that you seek your physician's guidance in choosing exercise that is suitable for your physical limitations. Those with heart disease will have particular restrictions. Those with lung impairment will have others. Again, the place to begin is with your life as it is now, your illness, your physical restrictions and abilities. Beginning again with regard to exercise involves mindful gentleness with a repairing body, not heroics to prove you are just like you used to be. Following the spirit of Benedict's Rule, we are best served by practice that is not harsh or burdensome.[1] Benedict, following St. Paul, recommends discipline for the body, a patient training through daily practice that takes individual circumstances into account.[2]

Much of what we see in magazines and on television leads us to think of exercise in terms of sports. Football, basketball, baseball, and soccer dominate the sports page. But exercise doesn't always involve sports of this sort. Most of us living with illness won't be able to participate in physical activities that over-stress the body. Instead, we are simply hoping to support the health and mobility that we still have. We need to be intentional about movement, about strength, about conditioning. Some of you will need to be involved in physical rehabilitation programs. Your physician should be able to guide you to programs that are appropriate to your needs. In larger cities, many hospital systems have wellness centers that include programs for patients recovering from surgery and who are recuperating from heart bypass. The goal is to honor your body, honor the life that you are presently living, by giving yourself the opportunity to support your own health in its present state.

Participating in the appropriate kind of exercise for your physical condition is a way of receiving the health you have been given, a means of expressing gratitude, and an act of faith in the God who is present within your very cells. In St. Paul's correspondence to the church in Corinth, he writes, "Or do you not know that your body is a temple of the Holy Spirit within you, which you have from God, and that you are not your own? For you were bought with a price; therefore glorify God in your body" (1 Corinthians 6:19–20). One way we glorify God in our bodies is by caring for them as God's own creation, sustained by divine mercy and goodness from moment to moment. This kind of care is not based in a desire to whip the body into an ideal physical state. Nor does it spring from a sense that driving the body harder is the way to get healthy.

Exercise that is right for your body, while living with illness, is an instrument of grace. It is a way for you to honor the life of God within you. When we begin to realize that our bodies are expressions of God's own creative work and that even when afflicted those bodies are continually engaged in myriad processes of transformation, we are less likely to treat the body with disdain or distrust. Pushing the body harder than is healthy and trying to whip it into an idealized state that it cannot attain are both unfair to yourself and your body, and do not honor the God who made you and loves you.

Discovering suitable exercise for you requires some discernment. You try some things and discover that they're not for you. Sometimes you'll push too hard and overtax your body and need to back off a bit. You will probably have days when the last thing you want to do is to think about exercise. Most of us do.

In beginning again, as you incorporate exercise into a rule of life for living with illness, remember that your body is a gift from God, even if your body isn't what it used to be. Remember to cherish the life that you now are living and to give support and nurture to yourself. Exercise is a way to *befriend* your body, to offer respect and dignity to your own flesh. So often we have been formed in such a way that we live in constant odds with our bodies. We may fret that we are not tall enough, strong enough, slender enough. Some of us were taught that our bodies were unwieldy or unacceptable—that is sometimes made worse by illness. If we hated our bodies before becoming ill, we may find that hatred deepening. We may harbor a sense of deep betrayal. "How could my body do this to me?" Carina asked of me. But over time, she began to see that it was not so much a matter of what her body had done to her, as it was a matter of her own neglect and harshness with her body that had depleted her strength and compromised her immune system.

Befriending the body involves learning to listen to the body. Exercise offers a way to become attuned to what the body is saying. It speaks its own language—sometimes in tight muscles, sometimes in a clenched stomach, sometimes in persistent aches. In times of illness, very short walks may be the most you can handle. And there may be days when bed rest is all that is possible. As strength returns, or as you become adjusted to a moderate level of exercise that works for your condition, practice noticing your body's responses to the exercise, and make adjustments accordingly.

After enduring several surgeries for a cardiovascular condition, an artist named Manuel said to me, "I have been taking these legs for granted for years. All these years I have been standing on them, walking on them. Never once have I said 'thank you' to the legs or to God. Now I am thanking these legs as my strength returns. Every day I am thanking them for holding me up, for letting me do my work, for taking me where I need to go." Manuel, in participating in his cardiac rehabilitation program, had begun to befriend his body, which he had formerly taken for granted. He had begun to literally step into gratitude instead of indifference or hostility. He could have stayed angry with his body for not continuing to operate without difficulty. However, as Manuel's strength returned, he found himself aware of his legs, aware in a way that permitted the intermittent pain of healing to serve as a trigger for offering thanks.

Walking

The simple activity of walking is a good, steady way to exercise, if your body can sustain the movement. Walking is also a fine way to pray. Walking meditation, done at a calm pace, matches breathing to your steps. Some of you may want to add a simple prayer to your walking. This could be a line of scripture: "You show me the path of life" (Psalm 16:11). Celtic Christians also had prayers that emphasize walking with Jesus. One such prayer follows:

> *My walk this day with God,*
> *My walk this day with Christ,*
> *My walk this day with Spirit,*
> *The Threefold all-kindly:*
> *Ho! Ho! Ho! The Threefold all-kindly.*[3]

This prayer has a good walking rhythm and a sprightly spirit. I have used it in my own walking and have found it to fit my own routine.

Of course, you can always create your own prayer. It could be something as simple as "Be with me." The point is to find a way to make the walking prayerful, rather than just a chore. The walking helps your body oxygenate, drawing the needed oxygen into tissues, breathing out the carbon dioxide. This process supports your body's healing and helps your tissues replenish needed stores of oxygen. Even if you are in the first stages of recovering from illness and are finding movement difficult, a walk around your living space is a way to begin.

You may find that you do not want to add a prayer of words. The simple fact of being able to move, able to walk, may be exactly the prayer that you need. As you walk and tend your breathing, you may find that the movement and the breath—the very fact that this is still possible—is prayer in and of itself. Pay attention to the way your foot touches the ground, to the heel and toes. Notice the rhythm and the connection.

However you pray in your walking, the essential thing is to pay attention and be aware of what you are experiencing. Know that the motion of your body is, in and of itself, a way to glorify God, a way to give thanks for this unique creation that houses your soul. Offer the walking as a time for gratitude, for enjoying the pace of your legs, for savoring the world you are walking in.

Stretching

Because I have scoliosis (a spinal curvature), I practice simple yoga stretches. I am not a yoga-adept person; however, the practice of stretching regularly, especially with an instructor who is trained to tailor the stretching to each person's needs, makes a big difference in flexibility. Many yoga instructors are well trained to help people who are living with illness. Most of the basic poses don't require exaggerated contortions; they simply help you lengthen your muscles. I always have a sense that my body is deeply content after a good session of yoga. I feel less kinked up or contracted, and my spine often feels more aligned and even somewhat lengthened.

Alejandra, who lives with a chronic lung disorder, has found that regular stretching and breathing also helps her avoid panic when she has difficulty breathing. The practice of tending to her breath has helped her to avoid holding her breath when she has a lung spasm. This gives her a sense of actively helping her lungs and her body and has helped with her own strength. As she breathes, she imagines the Spirit of God entering with each breath, circulating through her entire body, down to the tiniest cells. This practice has helped her to be more aware of God's presence with her and within her, particularly when her compromised lungs do not function well.

In addition, the stretching has helped Alejandra counteract her natural tendency to contract in response to the spasms. She stretches gently several times a day, even in the hospital. The longstanding practice of stretching and breathing is a foundational component of her own rule of life and has given her a way to actively pray with her body.

Other Forms of Exercise

Depending on what kind of illness you are living with, exercise may be imperative to well being. For those who live with diabetes or high cholesterol and heart problems, exercise is important for maintaining health. Avoiding exercise may even make your condition worse. Again, as you begin again it is always wise to consult with your physician. Some of you may be able to work out at a gym. Others may find that a program of regular swimming is the right choice for exercise. Try to discover what is best for your own health needs and then to allow that exercise to become a form of prayer. Enter the exercise with the desire to honor the sanctity of your own body and to nurture the life you have been given. Come to the exercise without heroic notions of being perfect. Seek to discover the right rhythm, the right form, the right pace for your own needs and for the ongoing care of your body. You may discover that you are capable of more movement and more flexibility than you would have expected. A good wellness center can be an ideal place to make these sorts of discoveries for your rule. Many of these centers and gyms offer the services of a personal trainer who can help you tailor a program that meets your needs and abilities.

I never would have guessed that I would relish both beginning Pilates (a form of body conditioning that emphasizes spinal and abdominal strengthening) and yoga as modes of offering prayer of and for the body, prayer to support living with illness and prayer of gratitude for ongoing—though very different—life. Pilates, yoga, and walking have given me appropriate ways to continue the befriending process with my body and to become more familiar with the language that this body speaks.

Questions for Reflection

1. What kind of exercise does your present physical condition permit? Check with your physician before beginning any program of exercise.

2. If you are already engaged in some sort of exercise, how do you feel about it? What kinds of thoughts and feelings do you have toward your body as you exercise? Could you transform these into prayer?

3. If you are fussing at your body during exercise, or feeling despondent over an inability to do as much as you like,

spend some time praying through those feelings. Be honest. Let yourself become aware of the kinds of animosity,
distrust, or unease you may feel toward your body. Are any
of these attitudes new? Or are they long-standing?

4. Psalm 139:13–14 says:

> I will thank you because I am marvelously made;
> your works are wonderful, and I know it well.
> My body was not hidden from you,
> while I was being made in secret
> and woven in the depths of the earth.

Notice the ways in which your body is marvelously made.
Give thanks for what you can do, even if you are not able
to do much in the way of exercise or do as much as you'd
like to do. Name the physical processes that allow you to
continue living. As you name each one, then pray, "Your
works are wonderful, and I know it well."

5. A process of befriending takes time and is grounded in
careful listening. How well have you befriended your
body? If this question sounds like something strange to
you, consider listening to your body. The next time you go
for a short walk, or stretch, or engage in whatever exercise
you are permitted, notice your body's responses. A friend
of mine who has a spinal distortion says that her body
always feels "glad" after doing some yoga. Another friend,
Robert, claims that when he does not walk it feels as if his
body is "sulking." These are examples of a process of
befriending, of listening, of beginning to notice that the
body is a gracious gift from God, worthy of respect and

kindness. Write down ways in which you become aware of your body's speaking as you exercise.

6. Draw a picture of the way you feel when you are walking. This is not intended to be a realistic diagram. This is an impression in color of your body when you are walking. As you choose colors, as you draw the impression, notice what occurs to you. Make notes after you have finished. Then sit silently in prayer. If drawing is not possible for you, try imagining the steps of this exercise. Picture your body walking or stretching. What colors do you associate with the movement? Do the colors intimate God's presence in the exercise, or your experience of divine support for your body?

Prayer

O God, in the course of this busy life give us times of refreshment and peace; and grant that we may so use our leisure to rebuild our bodies and renew our minds, that our spirits may be opened to the goodness of your creation; through Jesus Christ our Lord. Amen.[4]

7

Regimens of Medication and Treatment

"I hate taking these medications. I hate it. Every time I have to take them I am reminded that I am sick." That was how George started our conversation. An AIDS patient, George had lived longer than he ever expected to. He was able to continue living because of newly discovered treatments for AIDS. While he did not want to die, George also found himself feeling thoroughly antagonistic toward his medications. It felt as if the life that remained was completely enslaved to the daily schedule for taking the medications.

Most of us who live with chronic, progressive, or terminal forms of illness spend a lot of time with medications and treatments. One of the most obvious outward and visible signs of the ongoing presence of illness may be vials of medication on the kitchen counter or bathroom shelf. These bottles or syringes or bags of liquid medications tell us in no uncertain terms that the shape of our lives has changed. Initially, just remembering to take medications may be a big task, especially if you have an aversion to taking pills or medicines of any sort. Some readers may have to adapt to regular injections. Others may be receiving regular doses of chemotherapy or some other intravenous treatment that requires time and patience.

These medications and treatments, whether they are daily, weekly, or occasional, are also fruitful ground for your rule of life. First, it is imperative that you take the medications as prescribed. That is basic common sense. But it is also a form of obedience— not just obedience to your physician's orders, though it is that.

Benedict's perspectives on obedience help me when I have difficulty "following doctor's orders." In the Rule, Benedict links obedience intrinsically to humility. "The first step of humility is unhesitating obedience, which comes naturally to those who cherish Christ above all."[1] Obedience, humility, cherishing Christ—Benedict perceives that these attitudes are braided together. When I am listening to my body, to my doctor, and to the observations of family and friends, I recognize the limitations of my own stubborn reactions. I am reminded that living with illness connects me to a discerning community of friends, health care professionals, and family. I stumble into the goodness of humility that calls me into healthy relationship and honesty. Joan Chittister remarks, "Real obedience depends on waiting to listen to the voice of God in the human community."[2] The God who desires that we choose life offers us that opportunity through our acceptance of necessary medications, treatments, or injections. Benedict also counsels that nothing harsh or burdensome should be required in the life of the community. Consequently obedience is grounded in real trust—trust in my own awareness, trust in the guidance of physicians, trust in good friends.

This is obedience that involves listening. This listening is actually a deepening capacity to become attuned to God in and through all aspects of our lives, even in something that may seem as small and ordinary as taking prescribed medicines. (See chapter 9 for further discussion of obedience.)

When I first began taking various medications, particularly in those first years when it seemed overwhelming, I discovered that

I had to concentrate. I had to remember what I had taken when. I found myself asking my husband if he had seen me take a particular dose at a particular time. I was surprised that I could not seem to remember these important details. Finally I started making check lists for myself. I also purchased a pill-dispensing container that helped me keep track of what I'd taken and what needed to be taken still. While these strategies helped, they didn't banish the problem of forgetting. After months of this odd lack of focus, I realized that this inability to remember to take the medications might have something to do with my not wanting to face the fact of the illness. If I didn't take the medications, I wasn't sick—or so my behavior implied. It was as if I were trying to find a way to forget what had happened and to forget the needed changes in lifestyle.

In part, my lack of focus was due to simple fatigue and weakness. The longer it persisted, however, the more that lack of focus pointed to a real interior distress about being ill, a distress that was masked by external behaviors that looked like competence in handling all the changes. Rather than admit to that distress, I was telling family and friends that I was readily adapting, that the new routines weren't that hard, that it was all no big deal. My own deep unwillingness to form a habit of taking medication appeared to be rooted in unresolved sadness about the abrupt change caused by the pancreatic attack.

Some of you will not have had difficulties like this in adapting to regular regimens of medication and treatment. Others of you have struggled with your resistance and unease. Part of my own unease was also caused by not being sure about the long-term effects of the medications. Many of the participants in my classes have reported similar anxieties about medications, even when they are life-giving. In order to incorporate the taking of medications into your rule of life, you need to acknowledge your own underlying feelings and thoughts—whatever they are—about having to take regular medications.

It is helpful to be frank about any ambivalence you may have about your medications and to stay in regular conversation with your physician about that ambivalence. A doctor who truly cares about healing will want to hear what you have to say. If you notice problematic side effects, report them to your physician. It is helpful to the doctor if you keep a written log of when you take the medications and when the side effects show up. The more details the physician receives, the better able she will be to determine if something is awry. Of course, if a sudden allergic response of any kind shows up after you have started a medication, you should let your doctor know immediately and perhaps go to an emergency room.

Issues around medication are sometimes also linked to issues about authority—in this case the authority of the prescribing physician and the pharmacist. I have known people who just kept taking a medication without informing the physician of side effects because "the doctor told me to take it." That kind of response is not faithful to our bodies, to our physicians, or to the healing process. In fact, doing something like this shirks our responsibility to be a participant in our own care and nurture. Living with illness, really *living*, requires a growing maturity that accepts personal responsibility for the life we are still living. This growing maturity may manifest as an ability to be clear and forthright with doctors, rather than telling them what you think they want to hear. This maturity is definitely manifest as we practice taking medications and enduring treatments as a dimension of our rule of life.

I also know some people who have decided on their own, without consulting with the physician, to discontinue a particular medication. This, too, demonstrates a lack of communication and trust with the physician. Deciding to discontinue a medication without letting your physician know is a dangerous activity. At a minimum, you should check with the doctor's office to advise them of your decision.

Any rule, as I mentioned in chapter 2, is intended to put God at the center. When you are living with illness, it is easy to let the illness occupy center stage instead of God. It is easy to feel victimized by the need to take various medications or undergo treatments. It is important to refocus ourselves and look at these medicines and treatments as gifts from God. Consider the following as you live with medicines and treatments:

- We live in a time when a vast number of medications, both allopathic and homeopathic, are available to us.

- We are able to acquire the requisite medications when many people who need them either cannot afford them or live in countries where such medications are a complete luxury.

- The medications themselves connect us to a vast network of pharmacists, physicians, researchers, and chemists who are working to discover new ways of helping people who live with illness.

It may be helpful to regard the times of medication as a kind of daily office. Be prayerful in your approach to your medicines and treatments. If you have to take medications both in the morning and evening, for example, make those moments part of regular morning and evening prayers. At the very least, try to be thankful that you have the medicines you need and give thanks to God for them as you take them. You can also use your medication times as an opportunity for intercession. If you have to give yourself injections of insulin, you might consider praying for all others who suffer with diabetes as you give yourself the injection. If you are taking medication for high cholesterol, you could intercede for those who cannot afford those same pills. If you have arthritis and take anti-inflammatory drugs, you could call to mind all those with the same ailment whose impoverished status keeps them from having these medicines.

Having lived with a life-threatening lymphoma for several years, Bruce had to undergo radiation when lesions appeared in his brain. A nuclear physicist, Bruce approached his treatments from a perspective informed by his own scientific background and by the Gospel of John. Following the "I am" statements that Jesus makes in that gospel account, Bruce would enter the time of radiation repeating, "I am the light of the world" (John 8:12). Bruce discerned that the Light from which all creation springs dwelled both in the x-rays and in his own cancer-plagued brain. He regarded the treatments as revelations of God's light indwelling his body and his body dwelling in the Light. The treatments became an experience of mutual indwelling, of communion. Bruce began to also pray, "Abide in me as I abide in you," (John 15:4) sensing that the living Christ was communicating that in and through the radiation.

Taking a prayerful approach to the medicines and treatments we live with helps us include these necessary protocols under the canopy of grace, just like the other gifts of God we receive. This does not mean that taking medicines or dealing with uncomfortable procedures becomes a saccharine moment of happiness. Rather, taking a prayerful approach to your medical needs helps you grow in awareness that God is present even in this dimension of your life, and that these regimens are possible moments for communion in prayer and intercession for others.

Suggestions for Reflection

1. What kinds of medication do you normally take? How do you feel about regularly having to take prescribed medicines? If you are undergoing some kind of regular treatment, such as chemotherapy, how do you feel about your treatment? Make note of all the different feelings you may have, both comfortable and uncomfortable, positive and negative.

2. How do you pay for your medications? Do you have insurance? Are your medications more than you can presently afford? How does this affect you?

3. Practice adding intercessory prayers to your medical regime. These can be short and to the point: "For all of those who live with this same illness. For all of those who need these medicines and cannot acquire them. For all of those who brought this medicine into being." How does this practice affect your own experience of taking the medicines?

4. Some medications are literally taken by people all over the world (insulin, for example). Before taking your medication, allow yourself to pause and remember all the others who are connected to you in this way. Make note of your changing awareness as you practice this prayer of connection.

Prayer

Just to be is a blessing. Just to live is holy.[3]

PART III

PRACTICING STABILITY, OBEDIENCE,
CONVERSION, AND PRAYER

8
Stability

L iving with illness may offer you a peculiar gift. The jarring reality of a body afflicted with an ailment may wake you up from the narcotic habit of hurrying. Illness tends to make us stop, even when that's the last thing we feel like doing. In my own case, before I got sick, I enjoyed the variety of activities in which I was engaged. Such as? I had spoons stirring many pots, so to speak. To be stopped cold by acute pain and hospitalization was a very harsh awakening, but an awakening nonetheless. Once the initial shock and numbness abated, I began to realize how much I had overlooked in my life, how much I failed to see, perceive, and receive.

I would never have asked for the stability imposed by pancreatitis. Never. That said, I am grateful for the stability that illness forced on me. The illness sent me off to a monastic cell of sorts. My bedroom became my cell, the place where I lived. I prayed there. I rested there. I read and slept there. In those early months following the attack, it was tempting to imagine returning to a life that looked precisely like the one I had been living. I had, after all, enjoyed most of what I was doing. At the same time, this question began to haunt me: "How in the world did I do all of that? *Why* did I do all of that?" The bedroom had something to teach me. Since I couldn't get up and go to a meeting, or head to a class in graduate school, or prepare a confirmation class, I had to stay in my cell. I had to sit with my thoughts, my feelings, my own inner voices, and talk with them.

At this point, I decided to begin seeing a new spiritual director, a woman in her seventies. I knew for some reason that I needed an Amma (a spiritual mother) rather than an Abba (a spiritual father). I needed a wise woman to guide me through the illness, through the deep questions of midlife that were now elbowing their way into my awareness, through the sadness of watching my own mother weaken toward death. It is a good thing to have a spiritual friend or companion or director. During a time of illness, it is crucial. As illness leads you to sit in the cell, to be still, to be in solitude, you will need friends for the inner journey. I needed someone to help me hear what my soul was saying in the aftermath of the hospitalization. I wanted another pair of ears and another pair of eyes to help me hear and see what was emerging out of all that wreckage.

Benedictine Stability

In the context of the Benedictine Rule, the monk vowed to stay in the same monastic enclosure for his entire life, rather than rove around from monastery to monastery. Benedict lived in a time of social turmoil and violent upheaval. His insistence on a vow of stability offered hope and an opportunity to deepen and to grow. By staying in the same place for his vowed life, the monk made a profound commitment to love God and to love others. As each of us knows, learning to love within concrete circumstances is much harder than loving in romantic abstraction. When we commit to one another, to stay with each other in community, then we have to deal with each other's irritating little habits. One person talks with his mouth full. Another interrupts you every time you start to say something. Yet another tends to encroach on your personal space. We have to confront issues of shared labor and mutual care. But in exchange we are given the opportunity to truly know and love one another.

The roots of this vow of stability lie in the tradition of the Desert Fathers and Mothers of the fourth century. Their saying, "Go to your cell and your cell will teach you everything," sounds very countercultural in our society. We live in a time marked by mobility, by fast communication. We tend to move from one place to another, often because of changes in employment or because we receive orders to do so. We travel at high speeds— whether by car or train or plane. Rapid movement marks our lives. None of this is necessarily bad in and of itself. It can, how- ever, lead us to be so oriented toward whatever is next, toward the disappearing horizon of the future, that we completely over- look the present. We fail to be *in* our lives as we live them. We find ourselves, in the words of one Welsh poet, "hurrying on to a receding future."[1]

Stability, when living with illness, often takes the outward and visible shape of diminished physical activity. We can't hurry. The future is uncertain. Diminished activity often marks our lives. Stability may look like a different work schedule or no work at all. It may look like not being able to drive for some time. It may be marked by days of bed rest. But these inabilities or disabilities, be they permanent or temporary, are about becoming *stable.* In a medical situation, being "stable" is good news. When a patient's condition is "stable," at the very least it is not worsening. That moment of stability may be the much- needed pause in which your body can gather its defenses and begin to heal from within.

The word "stable" comes from a Latin root meaning "a stand- ing place," so when we are stable we are standing still. We aren't walking away from anything. We aren't walking toward any- thing. We are standing in a place that is our own, the place of liv- ing with illness.

Though it does not appear specifically in the scriptural narrative in Luke, Christian tradition has held that Jesus was born in a manger in a stable, the place where animals rest and feed. Many of the Christmas crèches that adorn our homes during the Advent and Christmas seasons depict the Holy Family in a lowly stable, with the baby Jesus in a manger. The stable of our body is precisely the place where new life may be born. The stable itself may be suffering from illness, yet within that space, when we are still and allow ourselves to wait, something new will come. This does not necessarily mean that we will be cured or that a terminal condition will miraculously disappear. The birthing of new life in the stable of illness is marked by deepening trust in God's mercy and presence, growing compassion for ourselves and for others, generosity of spirit and gratitude for life—even life that may be fading.

If you are living with illness, chances are that your body has already made you stop, or it is trying to do so. You've probably had to stop or adjust previous routines. Or perhaps you have attempted to maintain the same routine, while living with a new diagnosis. You are finding it increasingly difficult to maintain that pace. But living with illness almost always requires us to stop, or at least to slow down. Stopping and resting are the first steps toward recovering inward stability.

One of Benedict's great insights in a time of social upheaval was that a stable community offered the monk the opportunity to discover God's presence in daily living. Stability made it more likely that God's presence would be perceived in the regular, mundane encounters with others, in tending to each other's weakness. As Joan Chittister has observed, "Stability says that where I am is where God is for me. More than that, stability teaches that whatever the depth of the dullness or the difficulties around me, I can, if I will simply stay still enough of heart, find God in the midst of them."[2] Caroline, who lives with thrice-weekly kidney dialysis, has found that post-dialysis weakness forces her to be still for the rest of the day after receiving a treatment. With the help of her family, she created a prayer cell by obtaining a recliner and having it situated so that she could look out into her backyard. After treatment she rests, dozes, reads, and watches. Having been on dialysis for a couple of years, she has had the opportunity to gaze at her backyard regularly. This stability—which she certainly did not invite—has given her the gift of becoming attentive to the cycles of the season. She sees things she did not see before, such as the subtle shifting in color when autumn comes and the ruddy coloration of tree bark in early spring. In this stillness and stability, she has awakened to a sense of God's creative activity at work in her own backyard. She has come to know God's presence upholding her in the course of dialysis.

We resist stopping because often the moment we become still, we're besieged by inner desires, fears, voices, memories, or anxiety. Activity prevents us from having to deal with the distressing voices; stopping gives them an opportunity to speak. It is so tempting to flee from them. We can do that by resuming our activities, even when doing so harms us. Other times we flee the voices by actually feeding them with fantasies or fears or worst-case scenarios. Author Anne Lamott writes of her fears of having malignant melanoma in her book *Traveling Mercies*. Her father died of this cancer after it spread to his brain, and she fears the same fate. She gives us an honest, funny glimpse into her own turmoil after discovering she has a mole that needs to be biopsied: "That night at bedtime I looked down at my mole, and now instead of it looking like a small sow bug, it suddenly seemed to be alive and spreading, like a stain."[3] As Anne deals with the biopsy, she discovers that it helps to talk about it. She tells a woman at her church and another friend. She asks for prayers. And she begins to find a little stability in herself. The procedure occurs and she awaits the results. The mole is benign. "Sometimes

I found myself clutching the tender spot on my rib cage where the mole had been, cupping my hand over the two stitches like I was trying to keep my intestines from spilling out of the wound. But then I'd say to myself, 'I love you anyway, old thing.' And roll my eyes nicely."[4]

The story Lamott tells of her own coping with fear and biopsy gives us a hint for discovering internal stability for ourselves. None of us can ever stop the fearful thoughts and emotions that sweep through and shake us to the core. Anne recognizes her own tendency to expect the worst, to imagine dying before her time, to create scenarios in which she dies from the same metastatic melanoma that killed her father. Not only is she imagining the worst, but the fears take over her life, and she recognizes this. After several days of real fear, she heads to church and speaks all of this out loud. The minute she does that, it's not just roiling around inside her. Now all the fear and anxiety are in the lap of this kindly woman from her church, who immediately offers to pray. Anne's isolation has been transformed by the companionship of Marge. During the procedure, Lamott lets her doctor know—with characteristic humor—that she is scared. He assures her, matching the humor, that she will get lots of stickers for being brave. In other words, Lamott and her doctor find a way to bring the fear to speech.[5] Speaking the fear out loud diminishes the power of that fear, and stability comes in its place. One of the things I love about Anne Lamott is her complete honesty about her own inner struggle. She long ago ditched the need to pretend that everything is fine. And in that move, she stepped into funny, aching honesty. That is the beginning of inner stability.

Being honest, not taking yourself so seriously, helps you to seek a way out of the isolation of fear. When you allow yourself to be still, it's natural for worry, fear, and anxiety to present themselves. But you have choices about how you will respond to those feelings. Will you become the fear, or the worry, or the anxiety?

Or will you notice them, and ask for help? Will you identify completely with the fretting or will you recognize it for what it is, and ask a trusted friend to pray for you? The stability of the illness invites us to birth a new kind of vulnerability, something that our culture—sadly, even our churches—tends not to encourage or to model. Too often we associate asking for help with weakness or incompetence. If you ask another person to pray for you, you are tacitly admitting that you cannot do it on your own. If you pick up the phone and tell a friend that you are having a biopsy again and are terrified, you are choosing to be something other than the self-sufficient hero of your own script. As you live with illness, an inner stability begins to grow. This inner stability is marked by honesty, vulnerability, and a growing capacity for being direct rather than for playing games. Remember, Benedict guides us to see that humility, obedience, and cherishing Christ in ourselves and one another all go together.

In Anne's story, she reached out to two friends whom she could trust for good counsel and prayer. She recognized that she needed to find a way to ground her thoughts and emotions if she wanted to stop the inner whirlwind. Her friends gave her prayer and practical advice, which are often one and the same. Prayer does not always look like spoken words. (If you have made it this far in this book, you certainly are aware of that.) Prayer often looks like embodied response to another's need. As Anne had experienced the kindness of these two "midwives" who helped her birth new behavior, she discovered that action also led her to real gratitude to her own deep self: "I love you anyway, old thing." The inner stability allowed her to befriend her deeper self, the self that wasn't caught up in the vortex of fear. She discovered this person inside who asks the right people for help and has the wit to accept the help that is offered.

Stability allows us to stop, to have the humility to ask for help, and in so doing to drop any "I'm fine, thanks" persona. We discover the gift of vulnerability when we stop long enough to notice our defended behaviors and our various ways of being dishonest with ourselves, with one another, and with God. Author and retreat leader Esther de Waal writes, "I admit my limitations and my weakness, and I let someone else hold me up so that I can go on. This of course prevents any false self-image and cuts down my pride in my self-sufficiency."[6] So stability, through the practice of stopping and noticing and being honest, lets you meet this true self that is dwelling deep within you. Stability allows you to be your own best friend, to say with loving acceptance, "I love you anyway, old thing." Like Anne, you may say aloud after a particularly unnerving exam, "Thank you, thank you. I love you." This may sound narcissistic, but it isn't. An insidious and persistent rejection of ourselves so often plagues us when we live with illness. Some of you may even have picked up on subtle messages of rejection from nurses or doctors. I remember one physician in the emergency room who was clearly put off by the fact of my being sick in my stomach. (One wonders why he had chosen medicine as his profession.) In a tone bordering on disgust, the physician said to a nurse, "See that she gets help cleaning up." The nurse, on the other hand, was very kind. I was profoundly embarrassed by being sick in front of strangers, and the doctor's thinly veiled disgust didn't help me feel any better about myself.

You may have unwittingly accepted some rejecting stance toward your own body and soul. Practicing a kind of loving acceptance toward yourself, even vocalizing that in words of gratitude, can change these distorted perceptions. In writing about stability, Esther de Waal observes, "It [stability] means acceptance: acceptance of the totality of each man and woman as a whole person involving body, mind and spirit, each part worthy of respect, each part calling for due attention."[7] Your body, housing an illness, is worthy of respect. Your body, undergoing tests and other indignities, is calling for due attention. A rule of life for those of us living with illness includes a commitment to honoring our bodies and giving them respect.

De Waal goes on to say, "Only in our own day are we beginning again to discover that in our physical bodies we have a temple in which God can be reached, that the body commands respect and carries power, and that to deny this is to cut ourselves off from one of our most powerful sources of energy and strength on our way to God."[8] Your body, even when illness is your ever-present companion, is a temple, a sanctuary. We can't really run away from our illnesses. They live with us and we live with them. When you begin to regard the body you have been given in this way, you will begin to be knit back together, body, mind, and spirit.

Questions for Reflection

1. How do you honestly feel about your body? Are you feeling angry, sad, worried, upset? Try to name all of the different feelings that you may have about your body at this time.

2. What responses have others had to your illness? In what ways have you allowed these responses to color your own feelings toward your body?

3. How might you begin a practice of stability, of going beyond feelings of fear or anger or worry to a practice of honesty, vulnerability, and connection? Start noting ideas as they come to you.

4. Who could you turn to if you needed to ask for prayer? If no one comes to mind, remember that many churches keep prayer lists. You could call a local parish and ask to be put on their prayer list. In many cases, just giving your first name will be sufficient, should you wish to maintain some kind of anonymity.

5. How might you demonstrate increasing respect for your body? Be specific.

6. When you reflect on the "stable" of your own illness, what birthings of new life can you note? Sometimes these are very small moments easily overlooked, like tiny seeds that will soon burst. One way of practicing stability is to pay attention to those tiny changes, those movements toward love, joy, peace, patience, kindness, generosity, faithfulness, gentleness, and self-control (the fruits of the Holy Spirit, as listed in Galatians 5:22–23).

7. How have you begun to honor your body in the process of living with illness? If this is a new perspective for you, you might think in terms of how you think about your body, how you talk to yourself, how you pray about your body. It is helpful to start with what your body is accomplishing in spite of the illness—all of those organs and processes that continue to work. Give thanks for what is functioning well, and be mindful of ways in which to support your body.

8. This exercise requires the help of a friend and some butcher paper. Lie down on the butcher paper and have your friend trace the outline of your body. Then draw an image of new life growing within you. This could take whatever form or color you choose. Notice the color and the shape. When you are finished, offer this prayer, "In my body may I glorify God."

Prayer
The reason for stability? God is not elsewhere.[9]

9
Obedience

The word "obedience," in its Latin root, relates to hearing, to listening, to responding. I became very much aware of this when I took Maggie, my border collie, to puppy obedience class several years ago. We began with very simple commands, because she was only six months old and had a very short attention span. Maggie is bright, and she is also a herding dog. So while she might listen, she did not always respond to the commands as hoped. When I said "sit," sometimes she just looked at me and wagged her tail. Sometimes she ignored the command and did what she pleased, despite being offered a puppy treat to encourage her to follow through.

Maggie got better with consistent practice. She began to really listen. As she matured, I noticed that it was as though she were listening not only with her ears but with her whole body. She would change her body language, and she would almost anticipate each command (as any border collie owner will tell you, these are very smart dogs). Obedience began with wanting to listen. That was enhanced by her wanting to participate. The obedience was fully embodied when she responded with joy.

Some of you may have had the notion that obedience looks primarily like begrudgingly dutiful action. And I have had times in my own life when that was the only sort of obedience that I could muster. The Benedictine Rule, however, begins with the word "listen." Benedict invites us to recognize that we are in a relationship with God, and that if we never listen, we never offer God the opportunity to speak. If we never listen, we end up acting as if God is not present. If our prayer consists mostly of talking, talking, talking to God, it is akin to being in a one-sided conversation. As you know, those are not really conversations at all. Conversation is marked by mutuality, by a willingness to listen to one another, and by genuine respect and openness. Esther de Waal comments, "So to obey really meant to hear and then act upon what we have heard, or, in other words, to see that the listening achieves its aim. We are not being truly attentive unless we are prepared to act on what we hear."[1]

Obedience, then, is founded in relationship. As we come to know God's mercy and compassion, we will be given the courage to surface images of God that we have been hauling around since childhood—images that often look more like the Great Accountant in the Sky or the Crafter of Punishment. When I work with people who live with illness, I often discover that underneath fear and anxiety is a lurking suspicion that God chose to punish by bestowing illness. I always ask, "How does that God fit with a God who is willing to be born as a baby and die on a cross?" It seems to me that loving obedience cannot really take hold unless we have taken the time and the courage to really examine the false images of God that are unconsciously informing our behaviors. Stability, staying with ourselves, with our feelings and our fears, helps us to know what these false images might be. Once those false images are brought into the light, and are examined with a spiritual companion, they begin to lose their hold on our imaginations and our souls—and our bodies.

Julie, who lives with rheumatoid arthritis, said to me, "What did I do wrong that God did this to me?" That began an extended conversation about who God might be and who God is not. Julie had internalized her stern father's behavior and unconsciously equated that with God. This is not unusual. Most of us will discover that early in life we identified our parents with God and then began to attribute their behaviors to God. If you discover that something similar has been going on in your inner life, there is no need for self-judgment or self-criticism. Once you discover the real incongruity between whatever false images of God you may have (and we all have some) and the loving Mystery who brings all into being, redeeming and sanctifying the whole creation, you know the work you have been given to do.

Obedience begins in a patient sorting out of what is true and what is false. One aspect of that is to begin to discern who you really believe God to be. Inevitably that is intimately linked to discerning who you believe yourself to be. Illness may stop us in our tracks, and that stopping may save our lives. Once we stop, we can quit running, both inwardly and outwardly, from truth. I listen to many people who struggle with prayer and living with illness, with how to be faithful in the midst of harsh assaults on the body. In that listening, what I hear regularly is a sense that the illness has provided an unexpected (and often unwelcome) moment to let go of much that does not fit, does not feel true, does not have meaning. Fred, who suffered from heart disease, said to me, "I realized that I had been going so fast, I had been so intent on my career, that I had gotten hard. I don't want to end my life with this sort of track record."

Fred was learning to practice obedience. He was listening to his life and not liking what he heard. In that listening, despite the discomfort of coming to terms with some difficult truths about himself, he began to formulate a response. After a surgery, he felt he had received his life anew. He wanted to live in a different way. He, who had never allowed himself to be dependent upon anyone, had been forced to be dependent by virtue of his illness. He had to accept the ministrations of nurses, doctors, nurses' aides. He had to receive help to learn to walk again and to get through cardiac rehabilitation. In all of this, he was given a real gift. He was given the beginnings of humility.

Humility in Benedictine Tradition

In the Benedictine tradition, humility undergirds the life of the community. Humility is *not* humiliation. Benedict presents us with a twelve-rung "ladder of humility."[2] It appears in the middle of the Rule, indicating its importance. By addressing humility, Benedict is reminding us that we are always parts of the whole; we are not the whole. That may sound simplistic to you. However, our culture tends to form us in the mold of individualism and competition. Together, individualism and competition teach us to behave as if we do not need each other, as if each individual is a world unto himself. In stark contrast, religious tradition around the world affirms a completely different reality: we are each a part of an intricate, interdependent web of life that is not of our own making. You are a part of a beautiful, complex whole. Furthermore, the health of each part affects the health of the whole.

We know this also from St. Paul. In the correspondence to the church at Corinth, Paul uses the metaphor of the body to speak about the interdependence of members of the church. In giving the Corinthians this metaphor for the spiritual reality of the interdependence of the members of the Body of Christ, Paul asserts, "If one member suffers, all suffer together with it; if one member is honored, all rejoice together with it" (1 Corinthians 12:26). Implicit in Paul's teaching is the understanding that we have need of one another, and that we need to have enough humility to live from that awareness.

Another dimension to the Benedictine tradition of humility is that it leads us to continually sift through our behaviors, trying to become true to our inner life in Christ. This is not something that is done once and for all. This occurs only with patient daily practice. As we listen to and for God in the details of our lives, in the details of the illness, we will be listening for the truth in love. We will be listening within the context of our daily lives, in all of their singularity, for clues and intimations. Humility and obedience go hand in hand. One of the great graces of living with illness is that it may deliver you, quite unexpectedly, into gracious humility, into gratitude for your life, no matter how changed, and into an awareness that the world and God are very different from what you had surmised. You may discover in patient listening and obedient response that God is not the cause of your illness. You may encounter God present in and through the circumstances of the illness—in the doctor's office, in the treatment room, in the hospital, in the operating suite. As that divine Presence becomes more and more a felt awareness in your daily routine, you will be gently led to living in a way that honors that Presence—within yourself, within others, within every particle of matter that has been brought into being.

When living with illness, obedience comes with a particular kind of listening. We learn to listen to intuitions and promptings from within. Mattie, who had had a cancerous tumor removed some years earlier, had returned from travel abroad and noticed that she had a persistent pain in her side. Thinking she had probably pulled a muscle, she nevertheless kept having a feeling that she needed to see her doctor. After an exam that revealed nothing unusual, the doctor—who honored Mattie's own listening to her body—asked if she would mind having a CT scan. She agreed to the test. Several days later the doctor was calling to tell her that there was a tumor that needed to be removed. It appeared to have been caught early. The tumor turned out to be encapsulated and was removed without need for further treatment. When Mattie related this story to me, she pointed out that she kept having inner promptings to have the pain checked out. Her doctor also listened to those promptings. The end result was that a tumor was found at an early stage and removed. Mattie's willingness to listen, to be obedient in responding to those promptings, came from a habit of listening in prayer. Her first bout with cancer taught Mattie to slow down, to be still regularly, to listen to her body. Out of stability and obedience, she has learned to practice a patient and gentle listening with herself.

Diane, a friend of mine who coordinates pastoral care ministry in her parish, says that the kind of listening obedience that Mattie's story exemplifies is the same listening obedience we are called to when we receive those inner "nudges" to pray for someone else, to call another person on the phone, to write a note, to check on a neighbor. This is nothing less than listening obediently to the promptings of the Holy Spirit who moves within us with sighs too deep for words (Romans 8:26). This obedience is cooperative. When we listen in this way, we are acting to align our wills and actions with those of the living God. We are participating in God's active and embodied love, thereby honoring all of creation as God's own—even our bodies.

Following Instructions and Seeking Help

Obedience when living with illness also takes the downright practical form of following your doctor's instructions. This may mean incorporating a very different way of eating into your life. It may mean abstaining from behaviors that have imperiled your health. The taking of medications and following through with regular checkups are also part of this embodied obedient listening.

Since most of us could use some help as we seek to live faithfully with illness, one good practice is to take another person with you to crucial doctor's appointments. Particularly in the early stages of learning to live with illness, I found it very helpful for my husband to accompany me when I went to see the doctor. Doug would think of questions that I overlooked, and he would hear things that I was either too overwhelmed or too fatigued to hear. His listening with me helped form an obedience to the rule of recovering from acute pancreatitis. We were able to plan together and to reflect together as new information came forth, as medications were altered, as troublesome symptoms went undiagnosed. If you do not have a life partner who could accompany you to doctor's appointments, you could ask a good friend to be with you. Having two sets of ears doing the listening helps you hear the conversation with the doctor, receive what you hear, and respond with obedience by following instructions for the care of your body. At the risk of sounding too basic, I emphasize that this listening is enhanced when two are gathered together for the doctor's appointment.

Listening Obediently to Scripture: *Lectio Divina*

Lastly and most importantly, you need to be listening to scripture. In Benedictine tradition this is accomplished via a process called *lectio divina* or holy reading. (See my work *Broken Body, Healing Spirit: Lectio Divina and Living with Illness* for a full treatment of this practice.) Esther de Waal has remarked that Benedictine practice calls us to listen to scripture for strength as well as for knowledge.[3] *Lectio divina* involves several movements as we read scripture. It is, first and foremost, a listening for the Word of God within and through the words of scripture. *Lectio divina* offers the opportunity to listen for the Word speaking mysteriously to our own lives and circumstances. When we receive something so intimate and so personal, we are drawn again to love and drawn out of fear. We are called into relationship and out of isolation. We are moved toward trust and away from distrust. We desire to practice this kind of obedience, for in so doing we discover abundant life.

Lectio divina is a form of slowly reading "under the eye of God," waiting for a quickening of heart and listening for the stirring of the Holy Spirit. This is not at all like the reading you do for acquiring knowledge and expertise. You are invited to read scripture for formation rather than information. Using *lectio divina*, you will be listening deeply and responding creatively. For this practice, you will need to set time aside for a slow savoring of the Word. This is not meant to be done in a hurry, nor is it about reading a lot. For this practice you will need your Bible, your journal, perhaps some art supplies, and dedicated time and space. It will be helpful if you can set aside a time each day when you can be both attentive and relaxed.

The practice of *lectio divina* includes the following steps:

Silencio: The practice begins with recollection. Become aware of your breathing. You may need to stretch your body. Sit in a comfortable position. Let yourself rest in God. Breathe gently and deeply for several minutes before beginning to read. Allow yourself to let go of other concerns.

Lectio: Begin to read the assigned scripture slowly, savoring the words. You could follow the lessons appointed by a lectionary from your tradition, or you could simply choose to make your way slowly through the psalms or through another book of scripture. When a word or a phrase catches your attention, stop. Read no further. Let that word or phrase speak to you. Try to put the analytical mind aside and read from your heart.

Meditatio: Repeat the word or phrase that has caught the attention of your heart. (In the imagery from the Benedictine commentators, this is a form of "chewing," savoring, allowing yourself to receive the food of the scripture.) The repetition allows the attention to focus and permits a deepening of awareness. The repetition of the sacred words stirs memory, images, associations. Note these as they come up. If you find distracting thoughts coming up, gently bring your attention back to the word or phrase. If the thought is something you need to remember, jot it down, then return to your meditation.

Oratio: Let prayer form from the phrase or word that has been given to you. The prayer may begin with your own hopes, desires, needs, pains. Then let the prayer expand to encircle increasingly larger circles of connection. (For example, if you had been praying "For God alone my soul in silence waits" that could move to "I pray for all who wait for God—for those who make difficult decisions, for those who are in pain, for those who go without food, for those whose lives are in transition.")

You could let yourself use color and shape to respond in prayer. This might take the form of sketching, painting, making a collage. You may discover that the response is just color. Or you may discover one particular shape is linked to the prayer. This art response does not need to take a lot of time. The point is to allow color, shape, image, and line to be an integral part of your prayer, to offer a nonverbal, creative response.

Contemplatio: This last phase is a time for resting in God, for simply being still and letting the deep formation of the prayer continue.

Over time, practicing *lectio divina* regularly forms us. We allow the living Word of God to enter us, to speak in and through our lives, and to shape our prayer. When we enter this practice with honesty and humility, the listening that we bring to the practice leads us into gentle obedience. We discover that God is with us in the life with illness, and that therefore any aspect of that life may be an occasion for listening for divine guidance, instruction, or aid.

In addition, practicing *lectio divina* with scripture leads us to read the text of our lives. We may apply the process of *silencio, lectio, meditatio, oratio, contemplatio* to any occasion, any experience, any doctor's appointment, any treatment, any surgery—indeed, any aspect of living with illness. In so doing we begin to discover that these lives marked with illness are also holy scriptures, living narratives in which the God who sustains us seeks to offer us God's own mercy and compassion. As that awareness grows and deepens, we grow in mercy and compassion and are led, even sometimes when we are most in the throes of illness, to intercession and thanksgiving. This is not some "rose-colored glasses" perspective on life with illness. This is obedience in the midst of the details, an obedience that comes through stability, through listening and responding, through being humbled by the God who greets us in the operating room, in the lab, in the doctor's office.[4]

Suggestions for Reflection

1. When you reflect on the word "obedience," what comes to mind? Note memories, images, word associations, stories—whatever comes to your attention.

2. In your own words, being as honest as possible, describe God. This is for your own prayerful information; it is not a test of doctrine. As you begin to become aware of the images and impressions of God that you carry, you may want to explore some of them more fully.

3. Listening needs to be practiced. Spend ten minutes a day for a week listening to the sounds around you. Make notes of what you hear.

4. Listening is enhanced by silence. Allow yourself to give up an hour of television this week or to not listen to the radio while you are in the car. Notice what happens in the silence.

5. The phrase "listen to your body" may sound strange. You may begin to practice listening to your body by noting some of the following:

- When you are under stress, how does your body feel? Is the stress expressed in a particular organ or part of your body? (Does your stomach knot up? Does your breathing get shallow? Do your neck and shoulders tighten?)

- When you receive good or joyous news, how does your body respond?

- What signals does your body give you when you are fearful? Anxious? Worried? Sometimes our bodies know well before we register emotions cognitively. When we practice awareness of bodily response, we will be listening in a way that allows us to respond appropriately and prayerfully.

6. Obedience may be defined as acting on what we hear. For this reason obedience is the fruit of listening deeply, in humility. The response to this listening may take time to form. In fact, it tends to form over time rather than being impulsive. As you practice listening to your body, note what suggestions you receive. These may be corroborated by further listening, or they may not. Keeping a journal will help you discern a response.

7. Using the process of *lectio divina*, described on pp. 87–90, reflect on the following:

Return, O my soul, to your rest,
For the LORD has dealt bountifully with you.
For you have delivered my soul from death,
My eyes from tears, my feet from stumbling.
I walk before the LORD
in the land of the living. (Psalm 116:7–9)

As you read the verses, note what captures the "ear of your heart." Then repeat that phrase to yourself, noticing what associations come to you. Finally write out a prayer grounded in the meditation. If you wish, use these same verses for several days in a row.

Prayer

Day by day,
Dear Lord of thee three things I pray:
To see thee more clearly,
love thee more dearly,
follow thee more nearly,
day by day.
Amen.[5]

10
Ongoing Conversion

O ne of the mysterious paradoxes that Benedict learned from the writings of the Desert Fathers and Mothers was this: in the stability of the cell, and through listening with obedience, deep and real change transpired. The false life was replaced by a true one, formed by God. So the last of the three vows Benedictine monks and nuns take is one of *conversation morum*, or ongoing conversion. They vow to be open to God's transforming Spirit, to allow themselves to be changed. This same vow, coupled with stability and obedience, can help us to be continually and gently sculpted by the workings of God's love.

As we practice our rule, the promptings and intimations from the Holy Spirit help us to discard false behaviors and notions of ourselves and of God. As time passes, as obedience and stability grow within us, conversion occurs. God is the author of that conversion. When we notice and accept the invitation to participate in the conversion, we become co-creators, we allow ourselves to be made new. We become more likely to turn *toward* God rather than *away* from God. This is a movement of *teshuva*, the Hebrew word for return and repentance. Ruth Sohn, Jewish scripture scholar, notes, "The process of *teshuva* is often one of overcoming obstacles and feelings of hopelessness as we move slowly toward the hope of renewed life and redemption."[1] Those of us who live with illness confront obstacles and encounter sadness and despair. By practicing stability and obedience, which leads us into telling the truth, we practice *teshuva*, the ancient path of repentance and return, heading toward the Source from which we come.

As we enter into the holy conversation with the God who knit us together in our mother's womb, we also grow in humility, in that ability to take ourselves lightly and be more accepting of circumstances, of life, of God's own presence. I used to get disproportionately anxious about checkups. Finally my spiritual director counseled me: "Notice your actions. Then pray for help. Eventually you will begin catching the feeling before it becomes action. You will begin to notice it before the anxiety has you in its grip." Needless to say this required a lot of patience. I also had to learn to pay attention to the behaviors that told me I was really anxious. In all of this, my director kept encouraging me not to judge the anxiety, but to be kind to myself about its appearance, and to pray for assurance. So my prayer became a very simple one: "*Help!*" I wasn't used to asking for help, so this was a big step in honesty for me.

Once I'd learned to acknowledge my need for help with God, I was then able to start telling my husband and friends that I was scared. This was prompted by one friend asking straight out, "Is there anything you are afraid of?" Before I could formulate a response, I had tears in my eyes. It was as though the friend's question allowed the fear to come to the surface and be dealt with. Once the fear was spoken aloud (in this case a fear that there was some lurking malignancy, and that was the source of the continued weight loss), I felt a subtle inner shift. It was as if the poltergeist of unspoken fear had begun to leave the house of my soul. The odd thing was that the more often I brought the fear to speech with a few trusted friends, the less powerful its grip became.

I also began taking short walks to dissipate some of the anxiety. The prayer of simply offering the walk, offering the ability to move my legs, began to move into my life and into my body. The conversion—from frightened patient to a person who trusted that God was present—happened without any major plan on my part. In a bumbling way, I tried to follow God's lead by praying with and through the anxiety. There was, as my director pointed out, a sort of stability and obedience in that behavior. (She could be sort of sneaky in a holy way; she didn't point all of this out to me until after the fact.). And the tiny openings that allowed for deepening conversion to occur appeared almost without my knowing. For someone with lifelong scripts of being independent and competent, even admitting that the anxiety was in control was difficult. Asking for help was really new behavior.

Now, years later, I don't think twice about picking up the phone or sending an e-mail to several dear friends who are companions in prayer, soul friends. We pray regularly for one another and for the world. Simply making the phone call to ask for help changes my own internal reality. Sometimes a checkup is no big deal. Sometimes it is distressing. No matter what, I know I have friends who are with me in prayer.

When you live with illness, lots of changes get set in motion whether you like it or not. Frequently those changes aren't welcome. Yet you and your body are changed. How you respond to those changes is part of the process of ongoing conversion. Will you allow them to make you resentful and bitter? Will you allow sadness, grief, and anger to be honestly expressed, prayed through, and offered to God? Will you engage in the holy conversation with the living Word who is speaking through your life as you live with illness? Writing about ongoing conversion, Benedictine sister Joan Chittister remarks, "It is time to realize that it is not what happens to me in life that counts, it is what I do with what happens to me that is the measure of my happiness.

For some people, life is a challenge; for others, life is a continual crisis, the resolution of which is someone else's responsibility."[2] When I read these words in the context of living with illness, I discover that this Benedictine tradition of ongoing conversion offers a way to *live* with illness. Not to mark time, not to fall into dread, but a way to live.

It is not what happens to me that is the measure of my happiness. It is what I do with what happens to me. One of the obstacles you encounter when living with illness is the temptation to allow the illness to consume your entire identity. You become "heart disease" or "cancer" instead of Tom or Joan. Though the illness makes its own demands and requires certain actions from you, it will never be the sum total of your being. Only God in whom you live and move and have your being knows you completely. You may even be something of a mystery to yourself. As you begin to live with your illness as a rule of life, you will discover that your life is far more than an illness. You will discover interests, desires, hopes, and dreams that you didn't know you had. The paradox of illness, with all its limitations, is that living with it often provides us with opportunities to grow and to change. In writing to the church at Ephesus, St. Paul offered this prayer: "I pray that, according to the riches of his glory, he may grant that you may be strengthened in your inner being with power through his Spirit, and that Christ may dwell in your hearts through faith, as you are being rooted and grounded in love" (Ephesians 3:16–17). Living with illness invites us to pray that this Spirit of love will strengthen our inner being as well. This deepening spiritual vitality may occur in spite of physical distress, or perhaps even because of it. It is possible that even as the body fails, the inner being quickens and flames with love.

Carolyn, who lives with emphysema and is subject to regular bouts of hospitalization, decided that she has something to offer to others despite her condition. She and her dog began taking courses so that the dog, a fine Labrador retriever, could make nursing home visits. Carolyn (like me) learned some lessons about obedience in that training, and she also discovered that she needed to be able to offer something to other people. When she is able, she and the Labrador retriever make calls at a local nursing home. Carolyn reflected, "In the midst of my illness I found myself becoming more and more focused on myself. Some of that was necessary. But it also felt a little dangerous spiritually. It felt as if I wasn't connected to a larger life." As a result of living with illness, Carolyn realized that throughout her life she has practiced isolating behaviors, ones that were exacerbated by the emphysema. Seeing this, and responding by taking her dog to the nursing home to help others, was part of her conversion.

Letting Go and Openness

In reflecting on conversion and the Benedictine tradition, Esther de Waal states that this vow of conversion is a means of a constant letting go and of openness.[3] Living with illness is assuredly a means of teaching us to let go. At the end of our earthly lives, when we die and are received into the arms of mercy, we will have to let go of everything—our possessions, our bodies, our families, our landscapes, our earth-time. The vow of ongoing conversion invites us to practice this letting go so that inner transformation may occur, so that the inner being may be strengthened. We remain open to the possibility that God is slowly shaping us into the people we are called to be, and we acknowledge that there is much that we do not know or control.

Understanding and practicing this, like so many other parts of living with illness, is completely countercultural. Virtually nothing in our culture teaches us to practice this kind of openness, this kind of letting go. Rather, we are taught to be masters of our own destinies. We are encouraged to be "self-sufficient," whatever that means. We are taught to compete rather than ask for help. By a variety of means, we are led to practice acquisitive behaviors, succumbing to the insidious self-definition of "I am what I have." None of this opens us to ongoing conversion. None of this allows us to practice not being God.

Oddly enough, the illness you live with may be a kind of teacher. The illness may lead you to recognize a truth that the culture denies—that you are mortal and that one day you will die. Benedict counseled his monks, "Day by day remind yourself that you are going to die."[4] Benedict wasn't being morbid. His was a straightforward and realistic statement: we are all going to die. By being aware of that, we become more mindful that we are stewards of the life we have been given. Because being ill reminds us of our fragility and mortality, living with illness may be a peculiar means of grace. As you come to accept the fact of physical weakness, your whole world may look different to you. People who live with illness are less likely to take things for granted. Many of us who struggle with an illness take up that fine Benedictine practice of *savoring*—savoring your family, savoring your life, savoring the day. Illness can be a strong clarifier. The very fact of living with illness may provoke conversion in the sense that you find yourself suddenly open to awareness that is new and different. Old assumptions are jettisoned. Old habits are seen as they are: old and worn out. You may emerge into an inner space that has more breathing room. As the psalmist put it, you may discover, "He brought me out into a broad place; he delivered me, because he delighted in me" (Psalm 18:19).

Suggestions for Reflection

1. Ongoing conversion involves the practice of letting go. What has your illness caused you to let go?

2. Look at the list of things you've had to let go of and ask yourself if you need to be honest about grief for any of

these losses. If you discover grief is still with you, how might you gently address that grief?

3. As you review what you have let go, name each thing on your list and pray, "Into your hands, O Lord, I commend my spirit."

4. What are you discovering about your inner being as you live with illness? Spend some time praying these lines from Ephesians 3:16–17: "I pray that, according to the riches of his glory, he may grant that you may be strengthened in your inner being with power through his Spirit, and that Christ may dwell in your hearts through faith, as you are being rooted and grounded in love."

Practice this for a week, using the process of *lectio divina* described on pages 87–90. As you pray that your inner being may be strengthened by love, keep notes on your own responses and be mindful of any changes or conversions you experience.

5. In what ways do you need help? This could range from help with physical movement, to help understanding your illness, to help with depression. Become aware of the places in your life with illness where you need support. Begin to pray for guidance about who to ask for help, and then, when you are ready, ask for what you need.

6. For this exercise you will need a piece of clean paper (the bigger the better, but 8½" x 11" will do) and crayons or color markers. Make an outline drawing of your body. Don't worry about scale or doing this perfectly. Once the outline is done, color your body as you wish—without

regard for staying in the lines. In other words, color without fear of being graded.

Alternatively, instead of drawing, try this guided meditation. Lying on your back, begin to breathe gently and
deeply (if you cannot readily lie on your back, use a position that works best for you). As you breathe, focus your
awareness on the top of your head. Then gradually shift
the awareness to your face, your neck, your torso. As you
do so, pray, "Come, Holy Spirit." Notice any colors that
may come to you as you pay attention to your body. Do
any feelings or bodily responses show up? Notice and
make note. Once you have finished, pray the lines from
Ephesians 3:16–17 listed in #4 above.

Prayer
Come now reviving Spirit of God,
Breathe your healing strength upon those who suffer
And then, renew and bless all who
Proclaim and perform your liberating Word.[5]

11
Prayer and Living with Illness

When I was in my late twenties, the mother of two small sons, I began to feel an urgent desire for prayer. My friend Suzanne, also a mom with small children, gave me books on prayer—lots of books. I read Thomas Merton's *Seven Story Mountain* and *Seeds of Contemplation*. Then I started reading the English mystics—*The Cloud of Unknowing*, Julian of Norwich, Evelyn Underhill. Suzanne believed in starting with the best the tradition had to offer. Though I didn't always understand what I was reading, I did have the clear sense that this persistent desire for deep prayer was healthy and not neurotic. Many others throughout the ages (and later I found out, throughout all religious traditions) had been pulled toward prayer. I began to recognize there was healing medicine in these writings. I also discovered how important prayer is to my rule of life.

At the same time I was reading the gospels, and for the first time I was reading them through from beginning to end at one sitting. Perhaps because my children were small and that stage of motherhood requires keeping things simple, or perhaps because of Suzanne's good counsel, I began to understand that prayer wasn't just about words, prayer is a way of life. Prayer has helped me to stay sane over the years, especially when the demands of family and pets and work simply didn't allow for extended periods of quiet contemplation, of sitting still and listening for God's presence. Some days all I had the time and energy to do was mutter under my breath, "Give me eyes to see and ears to hear," but that was enough.

When you begin to understand that life and prayer are indissolubly joined, relying on technique or spiritual heroics fades in importance. The emphasis falls back to the place where Jesus put it—on the Great Commandments: "You shall love the Lord your God with all your heart, and with all your soul, and with all your strength, and with all your mind; and your neighbor as yourself" (Luke 10:27). Prayer that is grounded in these words—even the simple "Give me eyes to see and ears to hear"—is prayer that is embodied. Prayer begins to shape your life from the inside out. Body and soul are less separated as prayer becomes who you are and sinks into your very marrow. Silence, stillness, and solitude give the prayer opportunity to take root. Over time, the prayer becomes love in action. This kind of prayer is a lived response to God's presence and activity in the world, from the tiniest quark to the furthest galaxy. Prayer within a Benedictine perspective is grounded in the here and now, is open to new possibilities, and is genuinely honest in its expression. Prayer as a lived response is the goal toward which we live, the practice to which we aspire. It is also prayer that springs from real-life circumstance.

When you are adapting to living with illness, you may discover that the way you prayed before becoming ill simply doesn't work well any more. The illness has turned things topsy-turvy. You may still be in a state of numbness that precludes any real focus or concentration. Keeping in mind that praying and living go together, I offer these possible ways for beginning again with prayer.

Receiving Prayer

When illness has overtaken your life, you may be too tired or stressed or in too much pain to pray. This is a good time to practice receiving prayer even if you've never tried this before. To be the person for whom others are praying may be a new experience for you. Many of us have prayed for others, but knowing that friends and people who don't even know you are offering prayers on your behalf may be both a relief and a disconcerting reality. Being the object of other people's intercessions is a humbling experience.

If you feel uncomfortable about others praying for you, remember that intercession binds us together. Prayers for one another remind us that we all come from the same holy Source. Intercession is, at its root, a willing participation in the mystery of Christ's dying and rising, for in interceding we recognize God's infinite care for each person. We remember that God in Christ is doing better things than we could desire or pray for.

I am a member of a group in San Antonio known as the Tri Faith Dialogue. We are Muslims, Christians, and Jews who have been meeting together for the last four years to learn from each other and to grow in respect for one another's traditions and faiths. Last fall, when I fell ill again, I began to get e-mail correspondence from Muslim and Jewish members of the Tri Faith Dialogue, assuring me of their continued prayers for my healing. Some of these e-mails were from people I didn't even know. I had known real friendship in this group; receiving their prayers created bonds that were even stronger, more resilient than they had been. Later, when I met one Muslim woman who had prayed for me, the prayer had already begun to forge a friendship.

Joan Chittister writes, "To pray when we cannot is to let God be our prayer."[1] Receiving intercession, opening ourselves to the love and prayers of others, allows God to work within the human community. Let yourself know that others pray for you, that you are held up by intercession, that the prayers weave a strong web of connection that is in and of itself a prayer. In your fatigue, in your pain, in your deep uncertainty, your prayer may consist of simply growing in the awareness that others are praying for you. This is in fact letting go and opening—those two movements that allow conversion. It is letting go of thinking you can negotiate the illness without support. It is opening to the reality of being knit together, through Christ, to the community of those who pray for you.

Some Practical Suggestions

When praying while living with illness, forms of nonverbal prayer and of listening prayer may be especially helpful. In the paragraphs that follow, you will find a variety of ways to pray with and without words—using your hands, your eyes, your ears. By no means do I suggest that you do all of these. Rather, these methods are offered as possibilities from which you may choose something that fits your way of prayer as you negotiate life with illness. Some resources for further reading about many of these types of prayer can be found at the end of this book.

Prayer Beads

For centuries, people have prayed using aids for prayer. Prayer beads are one such aid. Prayer beads take a variety of forms. Some of you may pray with Rosary beads. Others may use the Anglican rosary. Some of you may have used Eastern Orthodox prayer beads. Holding and praying with beads reminds us that we have something to hold on to. When the press of illness and treatment threatens to overwhelm you, it may be helpful to carry prayer beads with you, especially into treatment and into the hospital. Holding the beads may be sufficient. Just having the tactile sensation of the beads in your hands may help you center. It may help you remember the prayers that others offer on your behalf. If you are able and desire to do so, say a prayer silently or aloud as you touch each bead. Simple prayers are best and easy to remember. You could pray, "Be with me," or "Stay with me." These evoke the story of the road to Emmaus in which the disciples ask the Risen Christ (whom they do not yet recognize as Jesus) to stay with them, for "it is almost evening" (Luke 24:29). They ask the Risen Christ to stay with them because they are uncertain, afraid, yet also encouraged by what he has been teaching them.

If you do not have prayer beads, you can find them at religious supply stores. You can also make them if you are led to do so. Picking out the beads, choosing color and shape and stone, can give you an opportunity to create prayer beads that are distinctly yours. Prayer beads are very portable, and they go readily to doctor's appointments, tests, labs, and hospitals. The constancy of the presence of the beads can be a reminder of the constant presence of God.

Icons

The Eastern Orthodox tradition of praying with icons has been very helpful to me in illness. An icon is a religious image that communicates Christian truth in visual form. The Orthodox tradition speaks of icons as being "written" rather than painted. An icon is understood as a sacramental word, a kind of word incarnate, that is "a door to eternity." The image is the outward and visible sign of spiritual truth. Gazing at an icon, you begin to see detail and line. As your eye begins to really see, the icon begins to teach you. Eastern Orthodox teaching tells us that icons both show us a person or event (such as the Crucifixion) and make the person or event a present reality. The visual language of icons imparts wisdom. As you behold the holy image, that image begins to shape the soul, to open you to love, to kindle the desire to be obedient. An icon may help strengthen inner stability, for the holy image feeds your soul, offering a kind of holy communion through loving gaze.

Traditionally, icons are accompanied by a small candle. My friend Susan, who is a member of an Eastern Orthodox church, keeps a small icon on a shelf in her dining area. When she is at home, a candle is lit before the icon, signifying the Light of Christ. If you are resting in bed a lot, you may want to place an icon so that it is readily visible. If you find yourself in a favorite comfortable chair for periods of prayer, you might want to set up a sacred space near the chair so that you can comfortably gaze at the icon.

You may find it helpful to play music such as Taize or Gregorian chant (see the section on music below) while you are practicing this kind of prayer with icons. Or you may discover that silence is more helpful as you watch the candlelight moving on the image.

Icons are available online and in religious bookstores. Praying with icons is especially helpful when you are living with illness, and particularly when you have reached a time where words no longer help. The image may be of Jesus, or of the Blessed Virgin and the Holy Child, or of a saint. There are many images from which to choose. When I taught a class on icons, I invited each participant to choose an image from an assortment of icon prayer cards I had obtained from a catalogue. I asked the participants to take their time and to spend the next week looking at the image that had entered their daily lives. The following week, we talked a bit about what had drawn each person to a particular image and what they had begun to see in the daily looking.

As the participants discussed their experiences, they realized that, in a way, they had begun a conversation with the image. It became apparent that each icon had its own meaning and value for the person who was using the icon for prayer. Over the following weeks, as each participant spent more time with the holy image, new meanings and insights emerged.

After three weeks, I invited them to choose new images. This time, someone said, "You mean let them choose us." In a way, this is true. The image may speak to something deep within your soul. I have one icon of the Annunciation to the Virgin Mary (Luke 1:26–38) that has been with me for eighteen years. Because it depicts the moment in which the Angel Gabriel says, "Do not be afraid" (Luke 1:30), I have used it when fear has stalked me. Icons allow us to pray with our eyes, and they open our eyes to prayer. This may be a way for you to enter prayer that sets aside the cognitive and analytical mind and allows you to simply rest in the gaze. As Henri Nouwen remarked, "Icons are painted to lead us into the inner room of prayer and bring us close to the heart of God."[2]

Music

When I was terribly weak, a friend of mine who has a large collection of classical CDs began lending them to me. My friend, a physician, seemed to be prescribing music almost as if it were a medicine. I had never prayed with music in this way. But as I listened, the music itself offered the prayer, even became the prayer. As many of you know, there are moments in the process of living with illness when the threads of your life are so unraveled it is hard to name what is happening. If you are also physically weakened, that makes verbal prayer even more difficult. Music, especially chant or classical music with no words, gives you a way to be borne up on sound. There is something primal about this practice, even when the music may be modern. The vibrations, the melody, the way in which the music swells and ebbs—all of these may give nonverbal sound to your prayer.

If you are unfamiliar with chant or classical music, you can always start with Gregorian chant or with music by J. S. Bach or Amadeus Mozart. These are tried and true choices. If you have a friend who is a musician, no doubt he or she would be willing to make suggestions.

When I first began to pray with music, the music was the prayer. For me, it was an experience of letting go and resting in the melody. I had a sense of the music supporting me, upholding me, and perhaps even helping me heal. I prefer to do less multi-processing these days, so I tend to listen to music when I am not doing anything else. You may find it helpful to listen to music while you gaze at an icon or read scripture. You may need to experiment to find what works best for you in your present physical condition.

Sometimes, in listening to music, you may find that thoughts, feelings, memories, or associations come to you. Just as with the practice of *lectio divina* (see pages 87–90), part of your prayer with music may be to gently tend these thoughts, feelings, memories, or associations. You may want to write about them. You may want to pray specifically about something that occurs to you.

For me, praying with music is a Sabbath practice in the sense that it has helped me to rest in God. I am not a musician, so I do not listen to music with technical or professional awareness. For some of you, music may offer a way to rest in the restorative presence of the God whose melody plays in us.

Set Time for Prayer

As you formulate a rhythm of prayer as a component of your rule of life, you may find it helpful to set aside dedicated time for prayer. Some of you will do this in the morning. Others will be more alert and open during evening hours. As I mentioned in chapter 7, it is possible to turn the schedule for medication into a prayer of the hours. This prayer marks times of day by daily regular times for reflection and scripture reading. Traditional Benedictine observance includes seven different daily times for prayer, plus a time for prayer in the middle of the night. But that kind of schedule would be hard for most of us to keep. Modern liturgical churches (Roman Catholic, Lutheran, Episcopal, and others) provide prayer forms for Morning Prayer, Noonday Prayer, Evening Prayer, and Compline (bedtime). Keeping some form of a prayer of the hours gives you a way to remember that each day belongs to God and to carry the day's concerns into prayer. (See the resource section for suggestions on books that are helpful in saying the daily office.)

If you are on a regular schedule for medication, this could be your "prompt" for keeping a prayer of the hours. Find simple prayers or create your own to say each time you take your medication. For example, in the morning, you could pray, "Create in me a clean heart, O God, and put a new and right spirit within me" (Psalm 51:10). You could follow this by saying the Lord's Prayer and asking for any intercessions that are on your heart and mind. If you have time, you could add scripture reading. Each time you take your medicine you could repeat a line from a psalm, add a prayer such as the Lord's Prayer or the Magnificat,[3] and include your intercessions. Traditionally, the different times of the day are linked with moments in the life of Jesus and in the liturgical cycle. A fine resource for helping you embrace this practice is *Praying the Hours* by Suzanne Guthrie.[4]

Centering Prayer

Springing from Benedictine tradition and from *The Cloud of Unknowing*, an anonymous fourteenth-century book on prayer, centering prayer is a straightforward, simple type of meditation. In this practice, you choose a word to repeat gently to yourself in prayer. The word could be "God" or "Friend" or "Jesus," or some other word that is sacred to you. Choose a word that has meaning and depth for you, a word that helps you remember that you are in the immediate presence of God. To practice centering prayer, sit in a comfortable but alert position. If this is not possible for you physically, choose a position in which your body is supported. If you are sitting, you may want to place your hands on your thighs, palms up, in a gesture of receptivity.

Then begin attending to your breath. First, notice your inhalation and exhalation. Then gently allow yourself to breathe a little more deeply with each inhalation. Don't force your breathing. Just let it become a little more natural and relaxed. As your breath settles into an easy rhythm, begin with a simple prayer of dedication. You could offer the Lord's Prayer, or a line from a psalm. I tend to use part of a hymn: "Come abide within me, let my soul like Mary's be thy earthly sanctuary."[5] Then begin to repeat silently to yourself the word you've chosen .

As you do this, you will find that your attention wanders. This happens to everyone who does centering prayer. As thoughts, or memories, or impressions come up, let them go and gently return to the repetition of the word. If you suddenly discover that you have gotten distracted and gone off with a stray thought, just let it go and come back to the repetition of the word. There is no need for irritation or frustration with yourself. If you find that your attention has gone from your word to something else, just direct the attention gently back to the word.

The practice of centering prayer allows us to begin to recognize that we are *not* our thoughts, we are *not* our emotions, we are *not* our memories. Over time, you begin to realize that there is a "you" who is beyond all of those thoughts. There is a "you" who is observing the thoughts, the memories, the emotions. You come to discover that you have a deeper self than you imagined. The practice of centering prayer helps us to practice letting go and being open. We learn to let go of ideas, opinions, and illusions. As we repeat our word prayerfully and in silence, the Holy Spirit bears witness that we are children of God (Romans 8:16), and all of our other roles and identities are revealed as partial. We learn to surrender all of those other identities and simply rest in God. This is an encounter of love; no explanations, no theories, no ideas are necessary. You allow the encounter to happen. Allow yourself to rest in the Mercy.

In *Finding Grace at the Center,* Thomas Keating writes of centering prayer, "The presence of God is like the atmosphere we breathe. You can have all you want of it as long as you do not try to take possession of it and hang on to it."[6] Centering prayer has the capacity to remind us that our center is in God, and that God is in our center. A deep refreshment of the spirit occurs when we allow ourselves to be in the presence of God who is always with us. In centering prayer we allow ourselves to remember God is eternally present with us, even when we forget.

Centering prayer is graciously portable. It can go with you into any circumstance into which the illness takes you. Practicing centering prayer is not magic. It is a means of learning to let go, to simply be with God, and let yourself be enfolded in mercy and grace. I wonder on occasion if centering prayer might be a good practice for dying. In dying, as we are born to eternal life, we will surrender all of our opinions, thoughts, and illusions. We will be in the presence of the living God who has knit us together, spoken us into being, crafted us with great care. That God, who in Christ has preceded us in death, will be with us in the final journey, and will receive us at the end.

Praying the Illness Itself

The illness itself also offers a place from which prayer may begin. By this I mean that the particular pain, treatment, or indignity that you endure with your illness is the place to start the prayer if you are willing to be honest with God. Tell God the truth in prayer about what you are experiencing. Speak what you feel, what you fear, what you hope for. The God "unto whom all hearts are open, all desires known and from whom no secrets are hid,"[7] awaits your trust. God patiently waits for us to speak what is on our hearts, rather than what we think God wants to hear. This practice of honesty goes back to stability, to standing within the reality of a body under duress. We pray from the reality of what we are living with, not from some idealized version of that reality. It also goes back to obedience, to that patient, deep listening that calls forth embodied response.

One of the richer aspects of prayer is that when you dare to speak what you need to say, you begin to be healed. By this I do not mean that you are magically cured of your illness. I mean that you make a choice not to put further energy into being someone you are not. You take the risk of faith, of speaking your self into being. In that moment, you step into an identity that is not as fragmented, not as split off from itself as before. Terry, a woman living with cancer, said to me, "Well, one good thing about this darn disease. I don't have the energy to play any games. I only have the energy to be me."

Philip, who suffers from a rare blood disorder, said that he always felt that he had to "dress up for God." "I felt like I was going to see someone who is very rich and powerful," says Philip of his former experiences. As a consequence, Philip's personal prayer was rather stiff and always formal. Philip said what he thought God wanted to hear. After becoming ill Philip began to try to be less formal. He began by just telling God about his day. As the story of the day unfolded, Philip discovered that he spoke more conversationally. He also discovered that after he had said what he needed to say, he fell into a contented silence. He simply sat and listened.

As he lives with his illness, Philip has learned to keep the conversation going, so to speak. He has also cultivated times of silence, times when he listens and waits and watches. For Philip, carrying prayer beads has been a means of being physically connected to his prayer. The weight and texture of the beads, which he normally handles every morning in prayer, helps remind him of God's presence when he is undergoing treatment.

Prayer in Worship

I've focused on personal forms of prayer up until now. Prayer with a worshipping community is also of vital importance when living with illness. If you are physically able, I encourage you to worship regularly with others. If a Sunday service is too hard for you to negotiate physically, try a midweek service. Participating in the worship of a community helps you stay connected to the larger community and to remember to pray for others. Being a part of a worshipping body helps you see beyond the boundaries of your own life, your own illness.

If you cannot attend church, there are a variety of ways to be a part of a worshipping community. If you were a member of a congregation before you became ill, you could ask for regular visits and, if it is your practice, for Holy Communion to be brought to you. In both Roman Catholic and Episcopal parishes, trained lay ministers are often readily available for bringing the church to you, so to speak.

There are also online resources for prayer and community. Here in San Antonio, many churches have websites, and some of them accept requests for intercessory prayer from those websites. Remember also that when you are hospitalized, most hospitals have chaplains who are on call twenty-four hours a day for pastoral care.

One friend of mine whose diminished lung capacity often prohibits coming to church has discovered a variety of ways to pray the daily office online. Grace Cathedral in San Francisco offers a spoken version of Morning and Evening Prayer. The Geranium Farm, a ministry of the Reverend Barbara Crafton, an

Episcopal priest, encourages participants to pray the office at home, and then signal that it has been accomplished by sending an e-mail message.[8]

At my Episcopal parish in San Antonio, on Wednesday we offer the Holy Eucharist with laying on of hands and unction. (Unction is a sacramental anointing with oil that that has been blessed. Prayers for healing are offered.) It is the custom on Wednesday night for those who desire to receive the laying on of hands and anointing to come to the altar rail. As each person kneels to ask for prayer, the others very gently lay hands on him. The celebrant prays the prayers for healing, laying hands on the head of the person asking for prayer. So, the person kneeling receives this gentle prayer of hands from others who are also ill. A tender silence surrounds the moment, marked by both respect and humility.

I have often thought that this service provides a glimpse of a beautiful reality. All of us are recognizing our own illness, and yet we are linked—as our hands portray—in praying for each other's well being. Some who have attended that service have died. Some have continued to live with cancer, diabetes, mental illness. Together the community prays and encourages each person along the way and occasionally celebrates both dying and rising.

Suggestions for Reflection

1. How are you currently keeping a time for prayer? Are you able to keep this time with some faithfulness?

2. Where do you regularly pray? If you don't have a space set aside for prayer, think about where that space might be. Choose a place (a chair, a room, a bed) that works for your physical condition. Pray in the same place regularly. This will allow the prayer to become a habit; once the habit is formed, the prayer space will call to you.

3. If you have a place for prayer, or if you are just deciding on one, what "vesting" might that space need to signal that it is set aside for prayer? This could be an icon, a candle, a Bible, or whatever might signal to you that this is a place for prayer. Spend some time thinking about this space and how it might be appointed for your prayer times.

4. Of the kinds of prayer presented in this chapter, choose one way of praying with which you have not had much practice. Try that practice for two weeks. Be patient and let the new way of prayer communicate with you. At the end of two weeks, reflect on what you have learned and what the process of that kind of prayer has been like. If you encountered resistance or unease, note that. If you found yourself content with the new form, then keep it up.

5. As stated earlier in this chapter, Joan Chittister has written, "To pray when we cannot is to let God be our prayer." When have you not been able to pray? What did you learn from those times? What did that feel like? In what ways did your sense of God's presence change as a result of not being able to pray?

6. Using your crayons or colored markers, draw your present prayer. Don't write any words. Simply offer your prayer in shape and color. Once the drawing is finished, sit quietly and listen. Finish with the Lord's Prayer. Alternatively, sit or lie in a comfortable position. Begin breathing slowly and gently. Imagine the shape and color of your prayer. Sit still and simply notice. Finish with the Lord's Prayer.

7. The Celtic Christian tradition offers a variety of prayers that begin "Bless to me."

One such prayer follows:

> Bless to me, O God,
> My soul and my body;
> Bless to me, O God,
> My belief and my condition;
> Bless to me, O God,
> My heart and my speech,
> And bless to me, O God,
> The handling of my hand."[9]

Using this prayer as a way to start, add a verse with particular reference to your body and your illness. For example, if I were to do this, I could add verses such as:

> Bless to me, O God,
> My weakened pancreas;
> Bless to me, O God,
> My energy and my stamina.

Create your own prayer, adding as many verses as you like, following the rhythm of the "Bless to me, O God" pattern.

Prayer

Be thou my vision, O Lord of my heart
All else be naught to me save that thou art
Thou my best thought by day or by night,
Waking or sleeping, thy presence my light.[10]

12

"I have no idea where I am going"

In the late 1970s, I began reading the works of Thomas Merton, prolific author and Trappist monk. As a Trappist, Merton followed the essentials of the Rule of St. Benedict. (Trappists keep a strict rule of silence while observing the vows of stability, obedience, and ongoing conversion.) Merton himself lived with a variety of physical ailments. His back was continually a problem. He had a variety of digestive troubles. As he aged, he experienced the aggravation of these and other physical distresses. Merton is best known for his teachings on prayer and solitude, though he covered a phenomenal variety of subjects in his writings. In all of this life as a hermit, a writer, a contemplative, a prophet, he lived with his illnesses and ailments. Those labels do not define him, though they were clearly one shaping force in his life.

One of Merton's prayers has been dear to me for a long time, especially so in the years since the pancreatic attacks. I cherish the prayer as a guideline for a rule of life, particularly for a rule of life when living with illness. With these words Thomas Merton offers a model of letting go and opening, of deep obedience, of stability grounded in the mercy of a loving and faithful God.

O Lord God,
I have no idea where I am going,
I do not see the road ahead of me,
I cannot know for certain where it will end.
Nor do I really know myself,
and the fact that I think
I am following Your will
does not mean that I am actually doing so.
But I believe
that the desire to please You
does in fact please You.
And I hope I have that desire
in all that I am doing.
I hope that I will never do anything
apart from that desire to please You.
And I know that if I do this
you will lead me by the right road,
though I may know nothing about it.
Therefore I will trust You always
though I may seem to be lost
and in the shadow of death.
I will not fear,
for You are ever with me,
and You will never leave me
to make my journey alone. Amen.[1]

In many ways living with illness does place us in the shadow of death. And a great unknowing comes with facing our own mortality. When we ponder the fact that our lives will end (though when and how are unknown to us), we find ourselves living from a very different reality, a very different context. During his time in the monastery, Merton discovered that God was "mercy within mercy within mercy."[2] Living with illness, as you begin to create a rule of life that is grounded in the reality of your day-to-day existence, you allow yourself to seek God where you *are*, not where you are not. This in and of itself is a mercy. You are not pretending that you are well. You are not diminishing the spiritual and physical effort involved in living with treatments or continued weakness. You are beginning again, with the flesh and blood of your body, to discern God's presence. Though you probably don't know what the road ahead of you holds, beginning with the desire to be with God, to please God, to seek God's mercy, transforms the way you walk with the illness.

Merton's prayer comes from a sense of deep trust in God's guidance and wisdom, the kind of trust we all need as we live with our ailments. So much of what we'd like to know or control isn't within our grasp. You may not know if you will find a way to live with your illness. You may not know what your life will look like as time goes by and the illness saps your physical strength. You may not be able to perceive a future of any sort. Into this unknowing, mercy comes. Mercy comes as we tend the details of nutrition, rest, exercise, and medications. Mercy comes as we allow ourselves to be shaped by the deep and prayerful listening of obedience, by stability marked by the willingness to stand in the reality of the illness, by choosing to be open, the willingness to let go, so that ongoing conversion may happen.

The practice of allowing the illness itself to be the ground for the rule is one of accepting the altered state of your life. To begin again, you first must recognize your life as it is presently configured. That recognition, that seeing, is the first step toward accepting. That acceptance allows you to befriend your present circumstances and to dwell in the present moment, even when that is difficult. There, in that present moment, God awaits you. God journeys with you in the shadow of death—death of old life, death of old identity, death of dreams. God delights in you and in your new beginning. You will find the divine presence in ways and places you never expected. You will discover in choosing to begin again that the possibilities for being made new come even at the lip of the grave. Even in the shadow of death, joy remains an incongruous possibility. Even in the shadow of death, God is with us.

Beginning again is the still point in the pattern of dying and rising. A holy pause exists before the dying turns to rising, a moment of choosing, perhaps as short as a breath, perhaps as long as a life. It is a moment of saying "yes," a moment of deciding that a life lived with God at the center might indeed be a life that is centered. It is a moment of knowing that though the particulars of your life are important, that they are not ultimate in importance. Choosing to begin again, to allow the illness to teach you how to shape a new rule for living in a God-ward direction, means opening to something new, something alive, something eternal. Whatever your illness, whatever the daily realities with which you live, in those details, in those difficulties and triumphs, the rule begins, and you begin again.

Notes for Creating a Rule of Life
for Living with Illness

1. List some of the "givens" with which you live. These would include dietary regimens and nutrition, rest, exercise, medications, physical impairment, etc.

2. Begin a list of what feeds your spirit. This could be anything from filling a bird feeder to reading, from taking a long, hot bath to getting a good night's sleep. Add to the list from time to time.

3. Include intentions for a regular rhythm of prayer and reading of scripture, making these appropriate to your physical condition. St. Benedict counsels that prayer should be short. You do not need to overburden yourself with a rigorous schedule. Offer what is appropriate for your capacity at the moment.

4. Begin to regularly include intercessions for others who live with your illness.

5. If you do not yet have an intentional relationship with someone who is a spiritual companion or spiritual friend, begin to pray about finding the right person with whom to begin that relationship. You may already know the person and only need to ask to add this dimension to your relationship. Having a companion with whom you can

talk honestly about the experience of living with illness and about your rule of life is healing in and of itself.

6. I have included updating information on my will, my medical directive, my durable power of attorney, and my living will in my rule of life. I see this as a matter of stewardship and as a courtesy to my family. I strongly recommend that if you have not taken care of these legal documents, that you do so. Be sure that those who care for you have been given clear instruction about your wishes, and that you have attended to the necessary details for disposition of goods and property.

7. I have also left written instructions for my funeral with my husband and my sister. These instructions include suggestions for hymns and lessons and instructions that I am to be cremated. Again, in the tradition of Benedict, this is a way of keeping death on my shoulder. This is not at all morbid. It is simply living with the reality of mortality. (In fact, I had many of these documents in place before the illness struck in 1995. A wise laywoman who was a nurse had convinced me at an early age to have those documents prepared, even though I was in good health at the time.)

Notes: _____

_____

_____

_____

_____

_____

_____

_____

Suggestions for Further Reading

Benedictine Spirituality and Rule of Life

Canham, Elizabeth J. *Heart Whispers: Benedictine Wisdom for Today.* Nashville: Upper Room Books, 1999. A delightful, engaging work that gives a realistic sense of Benedictine spirituality lived by people in the world.

Chittister, Joan. *Wisdom Distilled from the Daily.* San Francisco: HarperSanFrancisco, 1991. Chittister is a Benedictine; her text is strong, forthright, and directive. I regularly assign this text for classes on Benedictine spirituality.

de Waal, Esther. *Seeking God.* Collegeville, Minn.: Liturgical Press, 1984. This book is scholarly in an entirely approachable way and offers a variety of prayers and quotations from many sources.

Edwards, Tilden. *Living Simply through the Day.* Mahwah, N.J.: Paulist Press, 1998. Edwards's work is a fine aid for crafting a rule of life.

Farrington, Debra. *Living Faith Day by Day.* New York: Berkeley Publishing, 2000. This book is clear, succinct, and very helpful in understanding the components of a rule of life. It is also a fine text for use with a class, either in an academic or pastoral setting.

Guthrie, Suzanne. *Praying the Hours.* Boston: Cowley Press, 2000. Guthrie's reflections on praying the hours help us understand liturgical daily rhythms within the context of family, work, and church. The author is both poetic and humorous.

McQuiston, John. *Always We Begin Again: The Benedictine Way of Living.* Harrisburg, Pa.: Morehouse Publishing, 1996. This text is a good source for those who are just starting to read about Benedictine spirituality.

Palmer, Parker. *Let Your Life Speak: Listening for the Voice of Vocation.* San Francisco: Jossey-Bass, 2000. A Quaker, Palmer gives fine counsel with regard to vocation.

Ware, Corinne. *Saint Benedict on the Freeway.* Nashville: Abingdon Press, 2001. Ware's text is practical and down to earth, and she deftly relates Benedictine spirituality to daily life.

Sabbath and Rest

Heschel, Abraham Joshua. *The Sabbath.* New York: Noonday Press, 1979. A well-respected scholar and rabbi, Heschel offers the definitive Jewish writing on the Sabbath.

Muller, Wayne. *Sabbath: Finding Rest, Renewal and Delight in Our Busy Lives.* New York: Bantam, 1999. Muller's text could readily be used as a daily devotional or with a group. He brings to light many of our cultural attitudes and behaviors that keep us from observing Sabbath, while also offering remedies and suggestions.

Schaper, Donna. *Sabbath Sense: A Spiritual Antidote for the Overworked.* Philadelphia: Innisfree Press, 1997. Schaper's book is clear and funny, written from her own life context as a Christian clergy-woman married to a Jewish man.

———. *Sabbath Keeping.* Boston: Cowley Press, 1999. This text is more meditative in style. Some of the same material is found in *Sabbath Sense.*

Icons

Martin, Linette. *Sacred Doorways: A Beginner's Guide to Icons.* Brewster, Mass.: Paraclete Press, 2002. Intended for use by lay people who are not Eastern Orthodox, this book is an excellent introduction. The text includes historical information as well as theology and suggestions for practice.

Nouwen, Henri. *Behold the Beauty of the Lord: Praying with Icons.* Notre Dame, Ind.: Ave Maria Press, 1987. A beautiful little book that includes four-color reproductions of icons, Nouwen's work focuses on praying with the icons that accompany the text.

Prayer Beads

Hutson, Joan. *Praying with Sacred Beads.* Liguori, Miss.: Liguori/Triumph, 2000. This is a beginner's guide to praying with prayer beads.

Shannon, Maggie, and Eleanor Wiley. *A String and A Prayer: How to Make and Use Prayer Beads.* Boston: Red Wheel, 2002. This text is more eclectic in its approach than the one listed above; it also offers directions for making prayer beads.

Centering Prayer

Keating, Thomas. *Foundations for Centering Prayer.* New York: Continuum, 2002. This is a more comprehensive work that is the fruit of Keating's many years of teaching about centering prayer.

Pennington, M. Basil, Thomas Keating, and Thomas Clarke. *Finding Grace at the Center.* Woodstock, Vt.: Skylight Paths Publishing, 2002. This short group of essays is a basic introduction to centering prayer.

Prayers for a Daily Office

Newell, J. Philip. *Celtic Benediction: Morning and Night Prayer.* Grand Rapids, Mich.: Eerdmans, 2000. Newell's poetic prayers have an authentic, gracious feel to them. These are short offices that work well for those pressed for time.

———. *Celtic Prayers from Iona.* New York: Paulist Press, 1997. These prayers are inspired by those collected by Alexander Carmichael from the people of the Western Isles of Scotland. Again, the services are short, beautiful, and focused.

Saint Benedict's Prayer Book. York, England: Ambleforth Abbey Press, 1993. This prayer book includes services for morning, evening, and night as well as suggestions for praying the scriptures.

Tickle, Phyllis. *The Divine Hours Trilogy.* New York: Doubleday, 2000, 2001. In her comprehensive, imaginative collection arranged by the seasons of the year, Tickle draws on the Book of Common Prayer, the Bible, the writings of the early church, and other sources. This is a fine trilogy for personal prayer, though it may be more than a beginner would need. It is also a very good resource for teaching about fixed-hour prayer.

Notes

Chapter 1: Introduction

1. Joan Chittister, *Wisdom Distilled from the Daily* (San Francisco: HarperSanFrancisco, 1991), 7.

2. Ibid., 2.

Chapter 2: Rule of Life

1. *St. Benedict's Prayer Book for Beginners* (York, England: Ampleforth Abbey Press, 1993), 14. Also, The Rule of St. Benedict, 18:23, 73:8.

2. Timothy Fry, O.S.B., *The Rule of St. Benedict in English* (Collegeville, Minn.: Liturgical Press, 1982), 4:47, 28.

3. Ibid., Prologue 1, 15.

4. Parker Palmer, *Let Your Life Speak* (San Francisco: Jossey-Bass, 2000), 6.

5. Chittister, *Wisdom Distilled from the Daily*, 16.

6. Debra Farrington, *Living Faith Day by Day* (New York: Berkeley Publishing, 2000), 13–14.

7. *The Book of Alternative Services of the Anglican Church of Canada* (Toronto: Anglican Book Centre, 1985), 682.

Chapter 3: Dying and Rising

1. Naomi Shihab Nye, *Words Under the Words* (Portland, Oreg.: Eight Mountain Press, 1995), 29.

2. The Hymnal 1982 (New York: The Church Hymnal Corporation, 1982), hymn #516, v. 3.

3. The Book of Common Prayer (New York: The Church Hymnal Corporation, 1979), 306.

4. Ibid., 499.

5. Ibid., 504.

6. Ibid., 465.

7. Alexander Carmichael, ed., *Carmina Gadelica* (Hudson, N.Y.: Lindisfarne Press, 1992), 201.

Chapter 4: Nutrition and Mindful Eating

1. The Rule of St. Benedict, 39.
2. Ibid., 41:5.
3. Father John Guiliani in Marcia and Jack Kelly, eds., *100 Graces* (New York: Bell Tower, 1992), 22.

Chapter 5: Rest

1. Chittister, *Wisdom Distilled from the Daily*, 9.
2. Abraham Joshua Heschel, *The Sabbath* (New York: Noonday Press, 1975), 10.
3. Ibid., 74.
4. Donna Schaper, *Sabbath Sense* (Philadelphia: Innisfree Press, 1997), 20–28.
5. Heschel, *The Sabbath*, 30.
6. Chittister, *Wisdom Distilled from the Daily*, 163.
7. Henri Nouwen, *Lifesigns: Intimacy, Fecundity and Ecstasy in Christian Perspective* (New York: Doubleday, 1986), 60.
8. Ibid., 65.
9. The Book of Common Prayer, 134.
10. Ibid., 832.

Chapter 6: Exercise

1. The Rule of St. Benedict, Prologue, 46.
2. Ibid., 4:11.
3. Carmichael, *Carmina Gadelica*, 203.
4. *The Book of Alternative Services*, 679.

Chapter 7: Medication and Treatment

1. The Rule of St. Benedict, 5:1–2.
2. Joan Chittister, *The Rule of Benedict: Insights for the Ages* (New York: Crossroad, 1993), 59.
3. Abraham Joshua Heschel in *100 Graces*, 56.

Chapter 8: Stability

1. R. S. Thomas, *Laboratories of the Spirit* (New York: MacMillan, 1975), 60.
2. Chittister, *Wisdom Distilled from the Daily*, 15.
3. Anne Lamott, *Traveling Mercies: Some Thoughts on Faith* (New York: Random House, 1999), 179.
4. Ibid., 182.
5. Ibid.

6. Esther de Waal, *Seeking God* (Collegeville: The Liturgical Press, 1984), 33.

7. Ibid., 87.

8. Ibid.

9. Ibid., 65.

Chapter 9: Obedience

1. de Waal, *Seeking God*, 43–44.

2. The Rule of St. Benedict, 7.

3. de Waal, *Seeking God*, 33.

4. Certain material in this section published in *The Lutheran*, December 2003, vol. 16, no. 12, 24.

5. The Hymnal 1982, hymn #654.

Chapter 10: Ongoing Conversion

1. Ruth Sohn, "Verse by Verse," in Judith Kates, *Reading Ruth: Contemporary Women Reclaim a Sacred Story* (New York: Random House, 1994), 19.

2. Chittister, *Wisdom Distilled from the Daily*, 168.

3. de Waal, *Seeking God*, 70.

4. The Rule of St. Benedict, 4:47.

5. Frederica Harris Thompsett in Elizabeth Rankin Geitz et al, *Women's Uncommon Prayers* (Harrisburg, Pa.: Morehouse Publishing, 2000), 89.

Chapter 11: Prayer and Living with Illness

1. Chittister, *Wisdom Distilled from the Daily*, 32.

2. Henri Nouwen, *Behold the Beauty of the Lord: Praying with Icons* (Notre Dame, Ind.: Ave Maria Press, 1987), 14.

3. "Magnificat" refers to the song offered by Mary in response to the greeting of the Angel Gabriel (Luke 1:46–55). The text reads:

> "My soul magnifies the Lord,
> and my spirit rejoices in God my Savior,
> for he has looked with favor
> on the lowliness of his servant.
> Surely, from now on all generations
> Will call me blessed;
> For the Mighty One has done great things for me,
> And holy is his name.
> His mercy is for those who fear him

From generation to generation.
He has shown strength with his arm;
He has scattered the proud in the thoughts of their hearts.
He has brought down the powerful from their thrones,
And lifted up the lowly;
He has filled the hungry with good things,
And sent the rich away empty,
He has helped his servant Israel,
In remembrance of his mercy,
According to the promise he made to our ancestors,
To Abraham and to his descendants forever."

4. Suzanne Guthrie, *Praying the Hours* (Boston: Cowley Press, 2000).

5. The Hymnal 1982, hymn #475, v. 4.

6. Thomas Keating, Basil Pennington, and Thomas E. Clarke, *Finding Grace at the Center* (Still River, Mass.: St. Bede Publications, 1978), 30.

7. The Book of Common Prayer, 355.

8. You can register to be a part of this online network for praying the Daily Office by visiting Barbara Crafton's Geranium Farm website: www.geraniumfarm.org.

9. Carmichael, *Carmina Gadelica*, 197.

10. The Hymnal 1982, hymn #488, v. 1.

Chapter 12: "I have no idea where I am going"

1. Thomas Merton in *A Seven Day Journey with Thomas Merton* by Esther de Waal (Ann Arbor, Mich.: Servant Publications, 1992), 37–38.

2. Thomas Merton, *The Sign of Jonas* (Garden City, N.J.: Image Books, 1956), 351–52.